Technological Addictions

Technological Addictions

EDITED BY

Petros Levounis, M.D., M.A.
James Sherer, M.D.

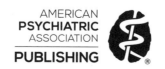

AMERICAN
PSYCHIATRIC
ASSOCIATION
PUBLISHING

If you wish to buy 50 or more copies of the same title, please go to www.appi.org/specialdiscounts for more information.

Copyright © 2022 American Psychiatric Association Publishing

ALL RIGHTS RESERVED

First Edition

Manufactured in the United States of America on acid-free paper
25 24 23 22 21   5 4 3 2 1

American Psychiatric Association Publishing
800 Maine Avenue SW, Suite 900
Washington, DC 20024-2812
www.appi.org

Library of Congress Cataloging-in-Publication Data
Names: Levounis, Petros, editor. | Sherer, James, editor. | American Psychiatric Association Publishing, issuing body.
Title: Technological addictions / edited by Petros Levounis, James Sherer.
Description: First edition. | Washington, DC : American Psychiatric Association Publishing, [2022] | Includes bibliographical references and index.
Identifiers: LCCN 2021017495 (print) | LCCN 2021017496 (ebook) | ISBN 9781615372935 (paperback ; alk. paper) | ISBN 9781615372942 (ebook)
Subjects: MESH: Internet Addiction Disorder | Behavior, Addictive
Classification: LCC RC569.5.I54 (print) | LCC RC569.5.I54 (ebook) | NLM WM 176 | DDC 616.85/84–dc23
LC record available at https://lccn.loc.gov/2021017495
LC ebook record available at https://lccn.loc.gov/2021017496

British Library Cataloguing in Publication Data
A CIP record is available from the British Library.

For Lukas and Shannon

Contents

Contributors

Muhammad Aadil, M.D.
Department of Psychiatry, Rutgers New Jersey Medical School, Newark, New Jersey

Lukman-Afis (Lukmon) Babajide, M.D.
Psychiatry Resident PGY-4, Rutgers New Jersey Medical School, Newark, New Jersey

Rafael Coira, M.D., J.D.
Child and Adolescent Psychiatry Fellow, New York Medical College, Behavioral Health Center, Valhalla, New York

Diego Garces Grosse, M.D.
Psychiatry Resident, Rutgers New Jersey Medical School, Newark, New Jersey

Faisal Kagadkar, M.D.
Resident Physician, Department of Psychiatry, Rutgers New Jersey Medical School, Newark, New Jersey

Yonatan Kaplan, M.D.
Department of Psychiatry, Rutgers New Jersey Medical School, Newark, New Jersey

Seyed Parham Khalili, M.D., MAPP
Clinical Assistant Professor, Department of Family Medicine, Keck School of Medicine of USC, Los Angeles, California

Petros Levounis, M.D., M.A.
Professor and Chair, Department of Psychiatry, Rutgers New Jersey Medical School; Chief of Service, University Hospital, Newark, New Jersey

Aitzaz Munir, M.D.
Department of Psychiatry, Rutgers New Jersey Medical School, Newark, New Jersey

Lancer Naghdechi, D.O.
Resident Physician, Department of Psychiatry, Rutgers New Jersey Medical School, Newark, New Jersey

Donya Nazery, D.O.
PGY-2 Resident, Department of Psychiatry, Rutgers New Jersey Medical School, Newark, New Jersey

Ana Claudia Zacarkim Pinheiro dos Santos, M.D.
Resident Physician, Department of Psychiatry, Rutgers New Jersey Medical School, Newark, New Jersey

Robert Rymowicz, D.O.
Fellow 2020–2021, Addiction Psychiatry, UCLA David Geffen School of Medicine, Los Angeles, California

James Sherer, M.D.
Chief Resident, Department of Psychiatry, Rutgers New Jersey Medical School, Newark, New Jersey

Heather Wurtz, M.D.
PGY-3 Resident, Department of Psychiatry, Rutgers New Jersey Medical School, Newark, New Jersey

Preface

Addiction to alcohol, tobacco, cocaine, and opioids can be devastating, as we all know. However, video games, online pornography, internet gaming, internet gambling, and other technological addictions can be every bit as addictive as substances. People have gotten so caught up in virtual pursuits that they have lost jobs, money, and loved ones in the real world. As technology becomes integrated into every facet of modern life, these technological addictions are becoming increasingly prevalent.

This book aims to help clinicians (as well as patients, parents, teachers, students, administrators, and anyone else who is interested in how humans interact with technology) master the fundamentals of the emerging technological addictions. The book is organized into 10 chapters: Video Games; Cybersex and Online Pornography; Internet Gambling; Texting, Emailing, and Other Online Messaging; Internet Surfing and Information Overload; Social Media; Online Shopping and Auctions; Children and Adolescents; Special Considerations for Older Adults; and New and Emerging Addictive Technologies. Some chapters overlap because people may be addicted to multiple technologies. Each chapter begins with the psychological and cultural context of that particular technology or population, which includes history and definitions, as well as the 21st-century reality of the people who struggle with these addictions every day. We also address the difference between healthy engagement with technology and addiction. Finally, each chapter includes some practice questions to cement the reader's knowledge and understanding.

Most of us know somebody, whether a patient, family member, or friend, who might be described as being addicted to technology. One of our patients, a 25-year-old man, could not date offline because he could not find anyone as attractive as his virtual partners. Another, a 20-something war veteran with schizoaffective disorder, ended up homeless because he racked up more than $10,000 in credit card debt buying virtual accessories to enhance his status in an online game. Yet another 20-something veteran with PTSD spent countless hours playing *Call of Duty*, exacerbating his symptoms to the point of requiring hospitalization.

Although these cases involve young, technology-savvy people, older adults are just as susceptible to the technological addictions. Older internet users who are less familiar with these technologies are, in fact, particularly vulnerable to scams such as the "wealthy prince" who happened to leave millions of dollars for them in his offshore bank account. Addiction to technology is non-discriminatory—anyone is susceptible. No preexisting psychological or physical conditions are required.

This is not to say that technology should be avoided. We do not advocate rolling back or restricting technology, which has become an increasingly beneficial and even necessary part of modern life. After all, there is little empirical data on this emerging problem, and the number of people who are technologically addicted make up a significantly small subset of the general population. However, we do want to alert the medical community and society at large to the addictive potential of technology and to the technological addictions as legitimate psychiatric conditions worthy of medical assessment, diagnosis, and treatment.

We would like to thank American Psychiatric Association Publishing for the opportunity to present this book to you and for providing space for these emerging topics. This book could not be possible without the dedication and passion of our coauthors, all of whom have treated patients with technological addictions and seen their devastating effects. We are also indebted to our patients, our mentors, and our students, who ignite our curiosity, keep us sharp, and motivate us to deepen our understanding and discover life-changing treatments.

Petros Levounis, M.D., M.A.
James Sherer, M.D.
Newark, New Jersey

CHAPTER ONE

Video Games

From Harmless Pastime to Internet Gaming Disorder

James Sherer, M.D.

In video games, you sometimes run into what they call a side quest, and if you don't manage to figure it out, you can usually just go back into the normal world of the game and continue on toward your objective. I felt like I couldn't find my way back to the world now: like I was somebody locked in a meaningless side quest, in a stuck screen.

John Darnielle

Culture, Psychology, and Popularization of Video Games

Addiction or Cure?

In May 2019, the World Health Organization (WHO) added gaming disorder (GD) to the 11th revision of the *International Classification of Diseases* (ICD-11), sparking controversy among mental health professionals and throughout the video game industry. Before then, gambling was the only behavior considered addictive enough to be listed in the ICD. Were video games as addictive as gambling? If so, did playing video games in excess truly qualify as a disorder?

The gaming industry's reaction was vociferous and swift. The Entertainment Software Association (ESA), the trade association for the video game industry in the United States, immediately fired back: "The World Health Organization knows that common sense and objective research prove video games are not addictive" (Gansner 2019). The ESA and its counterparts across the world highlighted research that contradicted the WHO (Przybylski and Orben 2018). Gamers and the gaming press questioned the WHO's decision, calling GD a "junk diagnosis" (Good 2019). YouTube personalities with tens of millions of active subscribers decried what they interpreted as the demonization of their hobby (Przybylski and Orben 2018).

Then, in March 2020, the WHO shocked everyone by appearing to reverse course—or, at the very least, to soften its rhetoric about the addictive potential of video games. In response to the COVID-19 pandemic, the WHO launched the "Play Apart Together" campaign, a global initiative to keep people at home, playing video games, to reduce their exposure to the virus. The video games industry, gaming press, and video game fans alike were reeling (Haasch 2020). First the medical establishment seemed to be branding gamers as addicts, then the were lauding gaming as a noble effort during an unprecedented pandemic—all within the span of a year. This seeming about-face by the WHO complicated an already difficult question: Are video games addictive and harmful, or are they just another pastime—and a relatively safe one at that? As with most addictive behaviors, the line between healthy engagement and dependence is a fine one. For video games, that line is constantly shifting as more research is done and popular opinion changes. Understanding video games as a cultural phenomenon and knowing their social importance along with their addictive qualities will help clinicians attain a well-rounded understanding of this nascent and rapidly expanding field of mental health.

A Cultural Phenomenon

Video games have come a long way since their origin in the latter half of the 20th century. In 1977, Atari made video games a household item with their Atari Video Computer System. Due to the popularity of games such as *Space Invaders*, along with the concomitant rise of arcades, Atari would go on to sell about 30 million units of their original console in the years to follow. Although that number seems impressive, it pales in comparison with the popularity of video games today. The Nintendo Entertainment System, released in 1985, sold more than 60 million units worldwide. In 2019, the game *Fortnite* sold 250 million copies. Perhaps "sold" is the wrong term because the base version of the game can be downloaded and played for free; *Fortnite*, like most modern games, is not confined to a console hooked up to a television screen. The same player can access their *Fortnite* account on their Nintendo system, their iPhone, their work computer, or practically anything with a screen. No matter where players access the game, their character and progress within the game goes with them. *Fortnite* is also a financial juggernaut, leading to $2.4 billion in revenue in 2018 alone (Shanley 2019).

How can a game that is given away for free make $2.4 billion in 1 year? It is estimated that about 69% of *Fortnite* players go on to make optional in-game purchases, averaging about $85 each (Batchelor 2018). This begs the question: Why pay for something when it is freely given away? Within games such as *Fortnite*, players can purchase in-game cosmetic items for their avatars via a randomized system commonly referred to as "loot boxes." The player pays for a set number of chances to receive rare items to show off to their friends. Loot boxes use variable-ratio scheduling to dole out rewards to players (Xiao 2018), and the odds of obtaining these items are not divulged to the player. In operant conditioning, variable-ratio scheduling creates a high, steady rate of response in subjects.

Aiming to make these optional purchases even more enticing, Activision, one of the largest video game publishers, has gone a step further. Activision patented a system that "matches an experienced player with a novice player to encourage the novice player to make purchases of items used by the experienced player. A novice player may wish to emulate the marquee player by obtaining weapons or other items used by the marquee player" (King et al. 2019, p. 134). Some players will go on to spend thousands in their quest to obtain the items of their choice. These players are commonly referred to within the video games industry as "whales," and much thought and effort is put into attracting them to the game (Iqbal 2018).

As video game industry revenue has exploded to overtake the film and television industries, games have evolved. When American gamers first met Super Mario in 1985, he was a two-dimensional representation made up of fewer than

200 pixels, or colored blocks. Back then, Mario could only do two things: run and jump across the screen. Players would pay once to obtain the game, with no additional purchases tied to the game after that. Today, vast game worlds are meticulously designed by teams of hundreds, if not thousands, of programmers, artists, engineers, and even behavioral scientists (Cuthbertson 2019). In addition to running and jumping, players can do anything from saving the universe to starting a virtual family. The financial cost of playing a game has become muddled by microtransactions facilitated by myriad new experiences made available to players. Game expansions, loot boxes, and other associated expenditures can mount quickly if the player wants to see all of the available content. A game listed for retail at $60 may eventually cost players hundreds, if not thousands, if they want to unlock all the game has to offer.

The Power of Escapism

What makes games so appealing? Why do many gamers prioritize them over family, friends, and their own physical and mental health? Video games offer a form of escapism steeped in immersion and wish fulfillment. When real life is harsh or bleak, games offer a gentler, more immediately satisfying alternative. As evidence of this, sales of video games during times of crisis skyrocket. At the height of the COVID-19 pandemic, sales of Nintendo's *Animal Crossing: New Horizons* shocked even Nintendo (Batchelor 2020). In *Animal Crossing*, players move to a utopia populated by anthropomorphized animals. Players build a dream home in an idyllic paradise, cultivate their island to their liking, spend time with their in-game neighbors, go fishing, and enjoy the sunset. It is a vacation that never has to end. In this world, there is no fighting, conflict, death, or disease. During the pandemic, many lamented the loss of simple daily routines to give life a sense of structure (Gottlieb 2020). *Animal Crossing* is tied to a real-time clock, so when it is morning in real life, it is morning in the game. The player and the characters have routines they follow from morning until night. Perhaps more than anything, this aspect of the game was greatly comforting to those mourning the loss of their previous daily habits.

The *Animal Crossing* series has always been moderately successful for Nintendo, but it has never matched the popularity of franchises such as *Super Mario Brothers* or *The Legend of Zelda*. However, when the newest installment of *Animal Crossing* was released in March 2020, the game was so critically acclaimed and financially successful that the Nintendo Switch consoles required to play the game became scarce. More than 11 million copies of the game were sold in less than 2 weeks, leading to more than half a billion U.S. dollars in revenue (Batchelor 2020). Everyone from television personalities such as Chrissy Teigen to politicians such as Alexandria Ocasio-Cortez were playing the game and speaking about their in-game experiences on social media. At a time in which many yearned for the return of normal life, *Animal Crossing* became a panacea. It offered players the opportunity to exercise agency and choice in a newly restrictive world. Adding to the game's success was its online functionality, which allowed players to visit friends' villages and spend time together in a virtual outdoor environment. It gave players access to the simple pleasures that life has to offer, pleasures that seemed so distant during the time of the pandemic.

Psychological Pull of Video Games

Although current events can significantly impact gamers' appetites, it does not take a pandemic to make video games alluring. Video games offer an opportunity for self-actualization that many crave, young and old alike (Przybylski et al. 2012). Being unhappy with one's age, height, weight, appearance, or sex is a foreign concept in virtual worlds with endless possibilities. Players can customize everything about their in-game avatars, from their eye color to their gender. The avatars that gamers pilot around virtual worlds often feel like a truer expression of self than is possible in the real world (Triberti et al. 2015). For children and adolescents, the opportunity to exert a level of agency typically reserved for adults is extraordinarily compelling.

Video games are designed to put players into a psychological "flow state" in which they are always challenged but never overwhelmed (Michailidis et al. 2018). While in this state, players face a challenge commensurate with their skill level. As their skill increases, so does the challenge. Video games dynamically change difficulty based on the player's performance. This encourages players to remain engaged for hours on end. In *Super Mario Odyssey* for the Nintendo Switch, if players die enough times, they are gifted an item that makes them nearly invincible. The players' frustration is thus placated, and they continue playing the game. The flow state is an inherently gratifying mental state, and one can easily imagine how players can lose hours of time in the blink of an eye (Velikovsky 2014).

The designers of *Halo*, a video game that helped launch Microsoft's Xbox console and would go on to sell tens of millions of copies, used these principles to their advantage. "In *Halo 1*, there was maybe 30 seconds of fun that happened over and over and over and over again. And so, if you can get 30 seconds of fun, you can pretty much stretch that out to be an entire game," one developer famously said (Kietzmann 2011). In such a loop, players complete tasks until they reach their goal, where they are met with fanfare and rewards. Then the player is given a new goal, and the cycle continues. This new goal may include some of the challenges the player surmounted in the previous level, with a few new ones peppered in. When surmounting these new challenges, the player is tested but never overwhelmed. This loop repeats even after the player beats the game.

Using new technologies and artificial intelligence, game designers can generate new loops *ad infinitum*. Games can be played indefinitely. At a certain point, developers begin to charge for additional loops, and players are willing to pay (Clark 2014). To design the most addictive loops, game studios have turned to the behavioral sciences. Studios such as Microsoft have hired mental health professionals to ensure a return on the sizable investment it takes to develop a game (American Psychological Association 2013). A modern marquee video game from an esteemed developer can cost hundreds of millions, or even billions, of U.S. dollars to develop. To help recoup those costs, developers collect biofeedback from quality assurance testers while games are being developed (Vincent 2018). They study the effect of reinforcement schedules on players' habits. They can identify which colors, sounds, and on-screen effects are likely to pique players' interest.

Addiction vs. Nonpathological Use

The popularity, accessibility, and wide variety of video games makes separating addiction from healthy enjoyment a challenge. Especially for parents with little or no knowledge of video games, the warning signs may be difficult to spot. Even mental health professionals disagree as to what qualifies as problematic usage when it comes to video games. After all, internet gaming disorder (IGD) is relatively new within the field of addiction psychiatry, and neither the definition nor the name itself are set in stone. Whereas DSM-5 (American Psychiatric Association 2013) refers to video game addiction as *internet gaming disorder*, ICD-10 calls it *gaming disorder*. The definitions are similar, but the diagnoses have a few key differences.

How Much Is Too Much?

Playing video games excessively is by no means exclusive to the younger population. However, most of the available research and data focus on adolescents. These studies are eye opening and have ramifications for adults as well.

How long, and how frequently, are children playing video games? How many hours per day is normal, and what should be considered excessive? For parents, these numbers can appear quite alarming. Playing time has quadrupled since the start of the 21st century (Rideout 2015). This is likely due both to the increasingly complex and addictive nature of games and to the exponential rise in their popularity. Of those who play video games, more than half play for >2 hours daily. Boys play longer than girls do, on average, but this is changing. Among the adult population, several studies suggest that women actually play more games and devote more time to games than men (Perrin 2018).

There is also a subset of children, 14% of boys and 5% of girls, who play video games anywhere from 4 to 10 hours a day. Parents do their best to limit children's screen time, but there is a large gap between the parents' perception of the number of hours their children are playing and what those same children report themselves (Alvord 2019). Most parents say curtailing their children's play time is an ongoing source of contention. A child who feigns sleep, only to sneak in some play time in the dead of night, is a common story.

This is especially concerning because all online habits, from video games to smartphone usage, have been shown to reduce subjective measures of mental health. The more hours spent gaming, the worse patients feel (Twenge et al. 2018). This is perhaps because video games can displace healthy behaviors. One's social life, academics, physical fitness, job performance, and sleep can all take a back seat to addictive video games. When new game consoles are released, time spent with friends and loved ones can decrease significantly. In 2007, when the original iPhone and the PlayStation 3 launched, the time that tenth graders spent with friends declined by as much as 15% (Twenge 2017). These same populations also reported feeling lonelier. Since then, these technologies have become more mainstream, and social well-being has declined.

DSM-5 Diagnosis

IGD is included in DSM-5 as a condition requiring further research. According to DSM-5, IGD is a pattern of behavior that causes significant distress or impairment. The condition is limited to playing video games and does not include problems with social media, online gambling, the internet, or smartphone usage. To meet the criteria for IGD, one must experience five of nine associated symptoms over a 1-year span. By requiring a relatively high number of associated symptoms, the authors ensured that IGD's prevalence would remain low. Therefore, a high degree of suspicion and significant impairment is required to diagnose it. Table 1–1 lists the associated symptoms along with some practical clinical advice for each.

ICD-10 Diagnosis

In contrast to the DSM-5 definition of IGD, the ICD-11 describes GD as a recurring behavioral pattern that involves impaired control over gaming, increasing priority given to gaming over other responsibilities, and continued play despite negative consequences. This behavior may be continuous,

TABLE 1–1.   Symptoms associated with internet gaming
                 disorder

Being preoccupied with video games	Given the ever-increasing popularity of video games and the expanding role they are playing in people's lives, preoccupation alone may be a less informative clinical indicator. For example, if a 14-year-old who is struggling in school plays video games for 5 hours nightly and 8 hours during the day on weekends, this would be deemed excessive. However, a 30-year-old employed as a game designer or streamer who plays the same amount may simply be doing so to maintain employment. If all or most of a patient's friends and social acquaintances are engrossed in the same game, cutting down on time played may be tantamount to spending less time with friends and family. Preoccupation must therefore be evaluated as going above and beyond what is acceptable for a patient's age range, social acquaintances, and profession.
Experiencing withdrawal symptoms when video games are inaccessible	Withdrawal symptoms from gaming present as emotional rather than physical; anger, irritability, depression, and despair are common. In children, poor impulse control may lead to tantrums and retaliatory behavior, making simply "cutting the cord" more complicated than it may seem.
Developing tolerance, or requiring more time playing video games to get the same satisfaction	Playing time increases must be compared with the patient's previous habits. For example, if a 17-year-old who is performing well in school goes from playing 2 hours to 3 hours nightly, this may not be a cause for concern. However, if a 15-year-old who is struggling in school goes from 10 minutes to 2 hours daily and only plays during class, this is clearly a cause for concern. Thinking in percentage increases rather than raw hour counts may be beneficial.
Being unable to cut down on playing video games despite efforts to do so	This can present in subtle ways. For example, if a player is unable to spend the desired time with one game, he or she may then spend more time with several different games, confusing the clinical picture and giving the clinician the false impression of improvement. Being thorough in taking the patient's history may reveal that the patient's seemingly reasonable enjoyment is more akin to dependence.

TABLE 1–1. Symptoms associated with internet gaming disorder *(continued)*

Giving up other activities to play games more frequently	Giving up other activities, such as sports or other hobbies, is perhaps one of the most concrete and useful symptoms for which a clinician can screen. Ensure that "spending time with friends" does not solely mean playing video games.
Continuing to play video games in excess despite obvious problems	A patient's own perception of impairment, just as with substance use disorder, may be compromised. This can lead to poor insight and the patient's inability to identify problems that others find obvious.
Deceiving family members about the amount of time spent gaming	Patients can go to great lengths to deceive family members. They may forgo sleep and play at night to give others the impression that they are gaming less. The financial costs of becoming truly engrossed in a game can skyrocket quickly, and patients may be deceptive regarding the amount of their income being spent on games.
Using gaming to relieve negative moods	Playing games to alleviate negative moods is perhaps less of a specific indicator because many, if not all, gamers would report that they use games to escape or at least to divert themselves from the struggles of everyday life. Even those with a healthy relationship with video games may report this effect to some extent.
Jeopardizing relationships or having lost a job due to gaming	Losing a job or experiencing a breakup because of gaming will be evident in the patient's history, but this particular symptom leads to a broader discussion. Many who enjoy games also seek to work in the gaming industry in some capacity. This industry has eclipsed film or television in terms of revenue, and hundreds of thousands of people are employed making games, so this is perhaps not as fantastical an ambition as one might think. Gamers are often fairly selective about choosing partners who also enjoy gaming. Therefore, behaviors that may have ruined a relationship may go unnoticed.

episodic, or recurrent, but it must be present for at least 12 months. Bipolar disorder and "hazardous gaming" must be ruled out before GD can be diagnosed. *Hazardous gaming* is a softened version of GD, defined as continued gaming despite some harmful consequences but without impaired control. ICD-11's definition of GD is clearly more inclusive than that of DSM-5's IGD, which has implications for clinicians practically and financially.

Prevalence, Comorbidities, and Risk Factors

How common is IGD? Prior to DSM-5's definition, the prevalence seemed almost too high to be believed. For example, in 2009, one study suggested that as much as 10% of the Chinese population and 9% of the U.S. population struggled with video game addiction (Fam 2018). After a definition was established, with its relatively high number of required symptoms, the prevalence decreased substantially. Around 0.3%–1% of the U.S. population is now estimated to meet the criteria for IGD. In certain Asian countries, the prevalence may be as high as 5.9% (Sussman et al. 2018). It is uncertain how the COVID-19 pandemic has affected rates of IGD, but if video game sales and social media engagement with games are any measure to go by, there will certainly be an increase.

Several comorbidities have been identified with IGD, including depressive disorders, anxiety disorders, and social anxiety (Liu et al. 2018). Other disorders (e.g., bipolar disorders, OCD, PTSD, substance use) are correlated with other technological addictions, such as problematic internet use, but not with IGD (Liu et al. 2018). Risk factors for IGD include male sex and having poor social skills (Rho et al. 2017). Several other risk factors are perhaps more subjective, such as having low life purpose, impulsivity, and poor emotional control; lacking parental supervision; and even having a poor relationship with one's father (Su et al. 2018). Given the variability in prevalence discussed earlier, it may also be possible that growing up in certain Asian countries, such as China or South Korea, may be a risk factor. In South Korea in particular, IGD has been labeled as the "number 1 public health threat," and there are laws that limit play, as well as hundreds of detoxification and rehabilitation residential facilities (Kelly 2014).

Positive Aspects of Gaming

A large amount of research and writing has shown that video games improve several aspects of our lives. Visual attention and tracking, as well as vision generally, can all improve with video game playing (Achtman et al. 2008).

Multitasking, hand-eye coordination, and the ability to rotate objects mentally in a three-dimensional space are tasks that get better with continued video game use (Ankay Yilbas et al. 2019). Providers should also consider that video games are a major avenue for normal socialization among youth (Lenhart 2015). Video games are designed to be social spaces in which players can meet up with friends, chat, and have fun, regardless of where they are. Especially during the COVID-19 pandemic, video games have been playing an ever-increasing role as social glue.

Being engaged with video games may also lead to employment opportunities (Molloy 2019). There are more than 2,400 companies in the gaming industry in the United States alone, employing more than 220,000 people (Takahashi 2017). There are also opportunities for those who want to cover the games industry for media outlets. With the rise of Twitch, a website where millions watch others play games, becoming a professional game streamer is also a potentially viable career choice.

Treatment

Although certain meta-analyses claim that no proven, evidence-based treatments for IGD are currently available given the small size (Zajac et al. 2017) and sometimes poor design (King et al. 2019) of existing studies in the literature, other researchers believe there is compelling early evidence for certain treatment methodologies. Regarding behavioral treatments, family-based approaches offer treatment advantages because parents and loved ones often require education about video games and the distinction between normal gaming and IGD. Family therapy that 1) encourages communication via active listening; 2) promotes establishment of time limits (including scheduled breaks from these rules and strict screen-free areas); and 3) focuses on the strengthening of family bonds can have a substantial impact on patients' lives (Han et al. 2012). On the other hand, boot-camp style programs are either ineffective or counterproductive (Zajac et al. 2017).

Cognitive-behavioral therapy (CBT) strategies and motivational interventions have been found useful (Greenfield 2018). CBT techniques specifically designed to treat internet addiction (CBT-IA), pioneered in 2013 by Kimberly Young, may improve outcomes in patients with IGD (Young 2011). These techniques focus on behavioral modification and cognitive restructuring and take a harm reduction approach, which is perhaps prudent when it comes to IGD, given the ubiquity of games and the difficulty of cutting patients off from them completely. However, research seems to indicate that standard CBT is just as effective for IGD as CBT-IA (Torres-Rodríguez et al. 2018).

Motivational interviewing has been shown to be effective for IGD (Kuss and Lopez-Fernandez 2016). Although patients have improved using motivational interviewing techniques, their progress may be somewhat slower compared with that of patients treated in CBT or with motivational interviewing plus pharmacotherapy. Another option that is available to providers is Naikan cognitive therapy, which has been well studied in relation to anxiety disorders (Nukina et al. 2005). This is a structured psychotherapeutic modality that seeks to help patients answer three questions related to their video game use:

1. Patients are asked what video games have given them, or how games have improved their lives.
2. Patients are encouraged to consider what they have given up in order to enjoy games.
3. Patients are encouraged to discuss what trouble video games may have caused in their lives.

Regarding psychopharmacological interventions, both bupropion and methylphenidate have been shown beneficial in relatively small studies (Han et al. 2010). Bupropion is perhaps the most studied medication for IGD, with success reported in various cases (Han and Renshaw 2012). In those studies, the side effects of methylphenidate often limited its use. In other studies, stimulants such as atomoxetine have been shown to be as effective as bupropion (Park et al. 2016). Additionally, given the numerous positive studies examining the use of opioid antagonists (e.g., naltrexone, nalmefene) in behavioral addictions, these medications may prove useful for IGD in the future (Bullock and Potenza 2012).

IGD is in its infancy as a diagnosis, which is reflected in the paucity of large-scale, robust, and reproducible studies currently available in the literature (Zajac et al. 2017). Inconsistent conceptualization of IGD may contribute to researchers' difficulties in designing and carrying out effective studies (King and Delfabbro 2014). The current definition is largely criticized for being too broad (González-Bueso et al. 2018). Adoption of a clear and distinct definition of IGD in the next iteration of DSM would be beneficial in this regard.

Special Considerations
Self-Expression and Self-Actualization

Perhaps unlike other addictive behaviors or substances, video games are a form of self-expression for many patients. Therefore, curtailing problematic behaviors may be interpreted by the patient as limiting freedom of expression or even infringing on their sense of self. By respecting patients' need for self-actualization, it is possible to help those who struggle with IGD to cut down on their use while still encouraging healthy engagement with the medium of video games.

Older Adults

Older generations of players are not immune to IGD (Bevans 2017). If patients have access to a smartphone, regardless of their age, they have access to a plethora of addictive games. It may be difficult for clinicians to identify dependence on games such as *Candy Crush*. These types of casual games receive less media attention than games such as *World of Warcraft*. Being detail oriented and asking patients to clearly monitor the time and money they spend playing can be helpful in differentiating healthy engagement from addiction.

Gaming and Socializing

Problematic gaming is associated with depressive disorders and anxiety disorders, especially social anxiety (Liu et al. 2018). It may be justified to explore a patient's social life in detail if you find the patient is relying more and more on games to foster friendships and spend time with others. On the other hand, games can be an appropriate and socially acceptable avenue for patients to find friends and practice social skills. Striking a healthy balance between socializing while playing video games and pursuing face-to-face interactions that works best for the patient is the goal.

Video Games History

When treating substance use disorders, taking a detailed substance use history is a key part of the initial interview. In a similar way, taking a thorough "video games history" can differentiate problematic use from normal play. By taking a chronological approach, mapping out patients' video game habits over time and correlating them with life events, clinicians can identify which games patients are struggling with. Like movies, video games exist as a vast media landscape, with genres that vary from fighting to exploration to simulation. A patient may easily become addicted to certain types of games while still being able to engage with others in a healthy and measured way. Here are some steps to consider when mapping out a patient's video games history:

1. Start with the earliest video games the patient can remember, even if those games were enjoyed primarily by watching another person play, such as a parent, sibling, or friend.

2. In addition to asking which games the patient plays, ask which consoles or electronic devices the patient plays them on. Games available on tablets and phones may have a higher addictive potential for some patients than games on a home console.
3. Record whether the patient plays alone or with others. As gaming becomes more socially acceptable, what may appear as problematic use may actually be healthy socialization.
4. Focus on the details of how the patient plays. How long does he or she play for, and at what time of day? What emotions does the patient say the game evokes?
5. Record appropriate life experiences and stressors to identify whether a traumatic experience led or is contributing to addictive behavior.
6. Record other hobbies the patient enjoyed at the time. If the patient can continue engaging in other activities and maintain relationships, IGD is less likely.

Table 1–2 presents a sample video games history. By chronologically mapping patients' use patterns, clinicians may find that certain games have been more problematic than others. Furthermore, such analysis may help guide psychosocial and pharmacological treatment options.

This video games history of the patient in Table 1–2 indicates that multiplayer online games such *World of Warcraft* and *Final Fantasy XIV* caused a decline in functioning. These games also led to a decline in the patient's other hobbies. The patient may be turning to this type of immersive game as a means of coping with deaths in the family. Other types of games did not have such a negative impact on the patient's life. Reduction or cessation of massively multiplayer online games is a prudent treatment goal. If patients are reluctant to give up gaming entirely, encouraging them to engage in other games that have less addictive potential may be a practical short-term treatment plan.

KEY POINTS

- In 2019, the World Health Organization classified gaming disorder in the ICD-10, and internet gaming disorder (IGD) has been described in DSM-5, making addiction to video games a diagnosable psychiatric disorder.

TABLE 1–2. Sample video games history

Date (age)	Games played	Played with others?	Details of play	Life events	Other hobbies
1991 (4 years)	*Super Mario World* (and other two-dimensional platformer/adventure games) on the Super Nintendo Entertainment System (home console)	Initially watched father play. Eventually played with friends but mostly alone.	Played for 1–2 hours at most, usually after school in the afternoon, as well as on weekends, four or five times a week.	Performing well in elementary school. Struggling somewhat with math but good grades overall.	Soccer, baseball, martial arts
1995 (8 years)	*Battle Arena Toshinden* (and other three-dimensional fighting games) on the Sony PlayStation (home console)	Played almost exclusively with father and very infrequently with friends.	Played after school or on weekends, for as much as 3–4 hours at a time, two or three times per week.	Strong performance in middle school. Expanding social group.	Soccer, baseball, martial arts, guitar, piano
2004 (17 years)	*World of Warcraft*, a massively multiplayer roleplaying game, played on both home desktop computer and laptop	Played with one friend patient knew prior to starting the game, as well as with a "guild" of friends met playing the game.	Played for anywhere from 6 to 12 hours daily after school, sometimes late into the night. Lost sleep frequently.	Lost a significant amount of weight. Death of grandfather.	Martial arts, guitar

TABLE 1–2. Sample video games history *(continued)*

Date (age)	Games played	Played with others?	Details of play	Life events	Other hobbies
2007 (20 years)	*Bioshock*, a story-driven first-person action/adventure game, played on the Microsoft Xbox 360 home console	Played with several college friends. Discussed game with high school friends over the phone frequently.	Played for about 2 hours at a time, generally late at night, but not impacting overall hours slept.	Excelling at college coursework, working part-time, large social group, relationship with girlfriend.	Martial arts, running, guitar
2020 (32 years)	*Final Fantasy XIV*, a massively multiplayer roleplaying game, played on home desktop computer as well as laptop	Played with a "guild" of friends met playing the game.	Played for anywhere from 8 to 16 hours daily after work, sometimes late into the night. Lost sleep frequently.	Lost job, broke up with girlfriend. Death of multiple family members.	Guitar (seldom)

- Many IGD symptoms mirror those of substance use disorders and other behavioral addictions.

- The rise of video games is causing an unprecedented shift in the way people engage with media and loved ones, and the prevalence of IGD may rise as a result.

- Behavioral techniques such as cognitive-behavioral therapy have shown efficacy in treating IGD.

- Medication such as bupropion and methylphenidate may aid in the treatment of IGD, but more research is needed.

Practice Questions

1. A 14-year-old boy with no past psychiatric history develops a habit of playing *Fortnite* 4–5 hours each day. He only plays after finishing his homework, but his gaming habit has started to negatively impact his sleep. The patient's parents become concerned and take him to see a mental health professional, who finds that the patient meets the criteria for internet gaming disorder (IGD). Which of the following psychiatric disorders is most likely to be present?

   A. Social anxiety disorder
   B. Borderline personality disorder
   C. Conduct disorder
   D. Intermittent explosive disorder
   E. Bipolar disorder

   Answer: A.

   Social anxiety disorder is often comorbid in patients with IGD, along with depressive disorders and other anxiety disorders. A link between IGD and borderline personality disorder (B) has not been identified. So far, there is no evidence linking IGD to conduct disorder (C). Although those who enjoy video games may be prone to impulsivity, intermittent explosive disorder (D) is not comorbid with IGD. Neither bipolar disorder (E) nor any disorder that may present with psychosis has been found to be comorbid with IGD.

2. A 23-year-old man with a past psychiatric history of major depressive disorder says his performance at work is declining. He recently broke up

with his girlfriend, is fairly isolated, and is spending an increasing amount of time playing *World of Warcraft*. He meets with a psychiatrist for the first time seeking medical treatment for both his IGD and his depression. His depressive symptoms include low energy, poor concentration, and overeating. He is not currently on any medications. Which of the following would be a good first choice for treatment in addition to cognitive-behavioral therapy?

A. Methylphenidate
B. Atomoxetine
C. Paroxetine
D. Bupropion
E. Lorazepam

Answer: D.

Bupropion, an antidepressant medication with uniquely activating qualities, has been shown to be efficacious in treating IGD, as well as depressive symptoms such as low energy and poor concentration. Methylphenidate (A) and atomoxetine (B) are also effective in treating IGD but are not approved by the FDA as monotherapy for depression. Neither lorazepam (E) nor any benzodiazepine has been shown to be an effective treatment for IGD. Paroxetine (C) is not the optimal choice due to its potential for causing sedation and possible drug-drug interactions.

3. The parents of a 9-year-old girl speak with her therapist about the increasing amount of time she spends playing *Animal Crossing*. She was given the game 2 months ago, and she now no longer enjoys playing soccer, her grades are suffering, and she has lost a concerning amount of weight. The parents insist that they are setting firm limits on playing time. Which of the following should the therapist tell her parents?

A. "It may be time to consider enrolling your daughter in a treatment facility because her behavior is worsening rapidly."
B. "I would advise you to unplug the Nintendo console from the television and hide the power cord at night so she cannot play past her bedtime."
C. "Many parents believe that they are setting strict limits on play time, but children often report the opposite. Have you considered using the parental controls on the game console?"

D. "In addition to cognitive-behavioral therapy, We should consider starting a medication, such as bupropion."

E. "Watchful waiting and behavioral monitoring are the best approaches at this time."

Answer: C.

Parents often believe they are setting strict limits on playing time, but children report the opposite. All major game consoles include some form of parental controls, which are more effective than verbal rule-setting alone. Boot camp–style treatment facilities (A) have not been shown to be as efficacious as other treatments. Simply "cutting the cord" (B) may be ineffective, especially with the Nintendo Switch, which can run in a portable mode off battery power alone. Starting bupropion (D) may be premature and could exacerbate weight loss. Although behavioral monitoring (E) may provide valuable clinical information, the patient is already experiencing detrimental symptoms. Using parental controls is a simple and risk-free method of addressing the problem, at least as a first step.

Resources for Clinicians, Patients, and Families

Entertainment Software Rating Board Tools for Parents (www.esrb.org/tools-for-parents): Provides free online tools for parents and clinicians who want to educate themselves about parental controls for gaming consoles. There is also a "discussion guide" with practical advice about regulating children's gaming habits.

Federal Trade Commission Resource on Kids, Parents, and Video Games (www.consumer.ftc.gov/articles/0270-kids-parents-and-video-games): Offers several web resources that can introduce parents and families to game ratings, parental controls, and the differences between games on consoles, on phones, and on the Web.

References

Achtman RL, Green CS, Bavelier D: Video games as a tool to train visual skills. Restor Neurol Neurosci 26(4–5):435–446, 2008 18997318

Alvord M: Digital Guidelines: Promoting Healthy Technology Use for Children. American Psychological Association, December 12, 2019. Available at: https://www.apa.org/topics/healthy-technology-use-children. Accessed April 9, 2020.

American Psychiatric Association: Diagnostic and Statistical Manual of Mental Disorders, 5th Edition. Arlington, VA, American Psychiatric Association, 2013

American Psychological Association: Dr. Tim Nichols, research psychologist. Careers in Psychiatry: Helping People Improve Their Lives. APA.org, 2013. Available at: https://www.apa.org/action/careers/improve-lives/tim-nichols. Accessed April 9, 2020.

Ankay Yilbas A, Canbay O, Akca B, et al: The effect of playing video games on fiberoptic intubation skills. Anaesth Crit Care Pain Med 38(4):341–345, 2019 30579943

Batchelor J: 69% of Fortnite players have bought in-game purchases, average spend is $85. GamesIndustry.Biz, June 27, 2018. Available at: https://www.gamesindustry.biz/articles/2018-06-27-69-percent-of-fortnite-players-have-bought-in-game-purchases-average-spend-is-usd85. Accessed April 9, 2020

Batchelor J: Animal Crossing is now the best-selling switch game of all time in japan. GamesIndustry.Biz, May 13, 2020. Available at: https://www.gamesindustry.biz/articles/2020-05-13-animal-crossing-new-horizons-has-become-the-best-selling-switch-game-of-all-time-in-japan. Accessed April 9, 2020.

Bevans A: Who plays mobile games? GamesIndustry.Biz, June 15, 2017. Available at: https://www.gamesindustry.biz/articles/2017-06-14-who-plays-mobile-games. Accessed April 9, 2020.

Bullock SA, Potenza MN: Pathological gambling: neuropsychopharmacology and treatment. Curr Psychopharmacol 1(1), 2012 24349964

Clark O: Games As A Service: How Free to Play Design Can Make Better Games. Boca Raton, FL, CRC Press, 2014

Cuthbertson A: Fortnite lawsuit: epic games hired psychologists to make game 'very, very addictive.' The Independent, October 7, 2019. Available at: https://www.independent.co.uk/life-style/gadgets-and-tech/gaming/fortnite-lawsuit-gaming-addiction-epic-games-a9146486.html. Accessed April 9, 2020.

Fam JY: Prevalence of internet gaming disorder in adolescents: a meta-analysis across three decades. Scand J Psychol 59(5):524–531, 2018 30004118

Gansner ME: Gaming addiction in ICD-11: issues and implications. Psychiatric Times, September 12, 2019. Available at: https://www.psychiatrictimes.com/article/gaming-addiction-icd-11-issues-and-implications. Accessed April 9, 2020.

González-Bueso V, Santamaría JJ, Fernández D, et al: Association between internet gaming disorder or pathological video-game use and comorbid psychopathology: a comprehensive review. Int J Environ Res Public Health 15(4):E668, 2018 29614059

Good OS: "Gaming disorder" officially on World Health Organization's list of diseases. Polygon, May 25, 2019. Available at: https://www.polygon.com/2019/5/25/18639893/gaming-disorder-addiction-world-health-organization-who-icd-11. Accessed April 9, 2020.

Gottlieb JF: The COVID-19 pandemic and emotional wellbeing: tips for healthy routines and rhythms during unpredictable times. Psychiatric Times, March 30, 2020. Available at: https://www.psychiatrictimes.com/article/covid-19-pandemic-and-emotional-wellbeing-tips-healthy-routines-and-rhythms-during. Accessed April 9, 2020.

Greenfield DN: Treatment considerations in internet and video game addiction: a qualitative discussion. Child Adolesc Psychiatr Clin N Am 27(2):327–344, 2018 29502754

Haasch P: Gaming companies are inserting WHO coronavirus guidance into games in an effort to encourage players to stay home. Insider, March 30, 2020. Available at: https://www.insider.com/play-apart-together-who-coronavirus-covid-19-blizzard-riot-twitch-2020–3. Accessed April 9, 2020.

Han DH, Renshaw PF: Bupropion in the treatment of problematic online game play in patients with major depressive disorder. J Psychopharmacol 26(5):689–696, 2012 21447539

Han DH, Hwang JW, Renshaw PF: Bupropion sustained release treatment decreases craving for video games and cue-induced brain activity in patients with internet video game addiction. Exp Clin Psychopharmacol 18(4):297–304, 2010 20695685

Han DH, Kim SM, Lee YS, Renshaw PF: The effect of family therapy on the changes in the severity of on-line game play and brain activity in adolescents with on-line game addiction. Psychiatry Res 202(2):126–131, 2012 22698763

Iqbal M: Fortnite usage and revenue statistics (2020). Business of Apps, November 28, 2018. Available at: https://www.businessofapps.com/data/fortnite-statistics. Accessed March 25, 2021.

Kelly RV: Massively Multiplayer Online Role-Playing Games: The People, the Addiction and the Playing Experience. Jefferson, NC, McFarland, 2014

Kietzmann L: Half-minute Halo: an interview with Jaime Griesemer. Engadget, July 14, 2011. Available at: https://www.engadget.com/2011–07–14-half-minute-halo-an-interview-with-jaime-griesemer.html. Accessed April 9, 2020.

King DL, Delfabbro PH: Internet gaming disorder treatment: a review of definitions of diagnosis and treatment outcome. J Clin Psychol 70(10):942–955, 2014 24752874

King DL, Delfabbro PH, Gainsbury SM, et al: Unfair play? Video games as exploitative monetized services: an examination of game patents from a consumer protection perspective. Comput Human Behav 101(December):131–143, 2019

Kuss DJ, Lopez-Fernandez O: Internet addiction and problematic internet use: a systematic review of clinical research. World J Psychiatry 6(1):143–176, 2016 27014605

Lenhart A: Video games are key elements in friendships for many boys. Pew Research Center: Internet and Tech (blog), August 6, 2015. Available at: https://www.pewresearch.org/internet/2015/08/06/chapter-3-video-games-are-key-elements-in-friendships-for-many-boys. Accessed April 9, 2020.

Liu L, Yao Y-W, Li CR, et al: The comorbidity between internet gaming disorder and depression: interrelationship and neural mechanisms. Front Psychiatry 9(April):154, 2018 29740358

Michailidis L, Balaguer-Ballester E, He X: Flow and immersion in video games: the aftermath of a conceptual challenge. Front Psychol 9:1682, 2018 30233477

Molloy D: How playing video games could get you a better job. BBC News, August 30, 2019. Available at: https://www.bbc.com/news/business-49317440. Accessed April 9, 2020.

Nukina S, Wang H, Kamei K, Kawahara R: [Intensive Naikan therapy for generalized anxiety disorder and panic disorder: clinical outcomes and background]. Seishin Shinkeigaku Zasshi 107(7):641–666, 2005 16146184

Park JH, Lee YS, Sohn JH, Han DH: Effectiveness of atomoxetine and methylphenidate for problematic online gaming in adolescents with attention deficit hyperactivity disorder. Hum Psychopharmacol 31(6):427–432, 2016 27859666

Perrin A: 5 facts about Americans and video games. Pew Research Center (blog), September 17, 2018. Available at: https://www.pewresearch.org/fact-tank/2018/09/17/5-facts-about-americans-and-video-games. Accessed April 9, 2020.

Przybylski A, Orben A: Why it's too soon to classify gaming addiction as a mental disorder. The Guardian, February 14, 2018. Available at: https://www.theguardian.com/science/head-quarters/2018/feb/14/gaming-addiction-as-a-mental-disorder-its-premature-to-pathologise-players. Accessed April 9, 2020.

Przybylski AK, Weinstein N, Murayama K, et al: The ideal self at play: the appeal of video games that let you be all you can be. Psychol Sci 23(1):69–76, 2012 22173739

Rho MJ, Lee H, Lee T-H, et al: Risk factors for internet gaming disorder: psychological factors and internet gaming characteristics. Int J Environ Res Public Health 15(1):E40, 2017 29280953

Rideout V: The Common Sense Census: Media Use by Tweens and Teens. San Francisco, CA, Common Sense Media, 2015

Shanley P: 'Fortnite' earned $2.4 billion in 2018. The Hollywood Reporter, January 16, 2019. Available at: https://www.hollywoodreporter.com/heat-vision/fortnite-earned-24-billion-2018-1176660. Accessed April 9, 2020.

Su B, Yu C, Zhang W, et al: Father-child longitudinal relationship: parental monitoring and internet gaming disorder in Chinese adolescents. Front Psychol 9:95, 2018 29467704

Sussman CJ, Harper JM, Stahl JL, Weigle P: Internet and video game addictions: diagnosis, epidemiology, and neurobiology. Child Adolesc Psychiatr Clin N Am 27(2):307–326, 2018 29502753

Takahashi D: The U.S. game industry has 2,457 companies supporting 220,000 jobs. VentureBeat (blog), February 14, 2017. Available at: https://venturebeat.com/2017/02/14/the-u-s-game-industry-has-2457-companies-supporting-220000-jobs. Accessed April 9, 2020.

Torres-Rodríguez A, Griffiths MD, Carbonell X, Oberst U: Treatment efficacy of a specialized psychotherapy program for internet gaming disorder. J Behav Addict 7(4):939–952, 2018 30427213

Triberti S, Serino S, Argenton L, Riva G: Being in an avatar: action and embodiment in a digital me. Stud Health Technol Inform 219:107–111, 2015 26799889

Twenge J: Have smartphones destroyed a generation? The Atlantic, September 1, 2017. Available at: https://www.theatlantic.com/magazine/archive/2017/09/has-the-smartphone-destroyed-a-generation/534198. Accessed April 9, 2020.

Twenge JM, Martin GN, Campbell WK: Decreases in psychological well-being among American adolescents after 2012 and links to screen time during the rise of smartphone technology. Emotion 18(6):765–780, 2018 29355336

Velikovsky JT: Flow theory, evolution and creativity: or, 'fun and games,' in IE2014: Proceedings of the 2014 Conference on Interactive Entertainment. Newcastle, NSW, Australia, Association for Computing Machinery, 2014, pp 1–10

Vincent B: This video game knows when you're scared—and it wants to use that against you. NBC News, August 26, 2018. Available at: https://www.nbcnews.com/tech/tech-news/video-game-knows-when-you-re-scared-it-wants-use-n903711. Accessed April 9, 2020.

Xiao L: Online gambling in video games: a case study on the regulation of loot boxes. Unpublished paper, 2018

Young KS: CBT-IA: the first treatment model for internet addiction. J Cogn Psychother 25(4):304–312, 2011

Zajac K, Ginley MK, Chang R, Petry NM: Treatments for Internet gaming disorder and internet addiction: a systematic review. Psychol Addict Behav 31(8):979–994, 2017 28921996

CHAPTER TWO

Cybersex and Online Pornography

Hacking the Human Sex Drive

Lancer Naghdechi, D.O.
Muhammad Aadil, M.D.
Faisal Kagadkar, M.D.
Petros Levounis, M.D., M.A.

Yeah. Not gonna lie. This sound [computer log-on chime] gets me hard…. I start off with some stills….Then…I start lookin' for a video….Once I [find one], goodbye. For the next few minutes, all the bullshit fades away and the only thing in the world is [porn] and that's it. I don't gotta say anything, I don't gotta do anything. I just fuckin' lose myself. There's only a few things I really care about in life. My body. My pad. My ride. My family. My church. My boys. My girls. My porn. I know, the last one sounds weird, but I'm just bein' honest. Nothin' else does it for me the same way, not even real [sex].

Jon Martello (Joseph Gordon-Levitt),
Don Jon *(film)*, *Voltage Pictures, 2013*

Culture, Psychology, and Practice of Cybersex and Online Pornography

The quote above is the opening line from the 2013 film *Don Jon*, written and directed by Joseph Gordon-Levitt, who also stars as the main character, Jon Martello, a young Italian American man living in present-day New Jersey. Jon lives a relatively normal life and considers himself a success—he is young, attractive, popular, financially stable, socially well connected, and has had no issues with his sexuality—except for his addiction to internet pornography, which ultimately ruins his relationship. This monologue gives insight into how cybersex may hijack our reward pathways and act as any other addictive substance would. We can see that Jon uses online pornography as an escape from his life. His experience is so euphoric that he prefers online sex to real sex. In the film, we learn that Jon spends a considerable amount of time watching and masturbating to online pornography despite his efforts and promises to stop and even after facing considerable negative consequences. He lies about his use and, when confronted, becomes irritated. Keeping Jon in mind, we begin this chapter with a brief history and some definitions, then we discuss diagnostic criteria, screening tools, associations, and treatments.

A Brief History of Pornography

The history of pornography is a long one, with the oldest known example being Venus of Hohle Fels, a 35,000-year-old, 6-cm sculpture of a woman with large breasts and visible vulva. Sex has always been a primary focus of art and a driver of social norms and taboos. Almost all forms of media throughout our history, from cave drawings and illustrated texts to photographs and films, have been used in some erotic or pornographic fashion. Fast forward to 1896, when the first erotic film, titled *Le Coucher de la Mariée* (a striptease), was released (Raustiala and Sprigman 2018). Pornography—and human sexuality as a whole—has never been the same.

Pornography is no longer just a box of videotapes in the attic or a pile of magazines stashed under a mattress. Except for the photograph, the internet is perhaps the single most important driving force for the advancement and distribution of pornography. It has transformed pornography into an "all you can consume" entity with an infinite supply of content, performers, and genres. In the past few decades, the introduction of the smartphone has added to the internet's already long reach, bringing access to pornography to almost anyone.

Online pornography has become a multibillion-dollar industry. Mindgeek, self-described as an information technology firm, is the little-known parent company of several well-known and heavily trafficked pornography sites such as Pornhub, YouPorn, GayTube, Brazzers, and Digital Playground. Its main competitor, WGCZ Holdings, hosts XVideos and Bang Bros, among many others. In 2015, Mindgeek alone was estimated to make about $100 billion in global revenue per year, more than double the $38 billion global box office revenue of motion pictures in 2016 (Raustiala and Sprigman 2018).

According to data published on Pornhub (www.pornhub.com/insights), in 2019 there were 42 billion total visits to its site, averaging 115 million daily visits. That year, 1.36 million hours (169 years) of new content was uploaded. The average time spent on Pornhub was 10.5 minutes. Pornhub is also used as a social media platform, as evidenced by the 70 million messages sent between users and 11.5 million comments on its videos in 2019 alone. More than three-quarters of users (77%) accessed the site on their smartphones, an increase of 7% over 2018. The data also show that users are predominantly men, with women comprising 32% of visitors, an increase of 3% from 2018. The average age of users was 36 years, with those ages 18–30 making up more than 60% of traffic (Silver 2019).

So powerful is the pornography industry that it has influenced technology, politics, public health, and overall society. It has driven markets in favor of one type of media over another. Examples include digital cameras (vs. film), VHS (vs. Betamax), and Blu-Ray DVD (vs. HD DVD). In these cases, the pornography industry chose which format held *more* content, as opposed to the quality of the content (Glass 2014; Raustiala and Sprigman 2018). The industry also has its own lobby, called the Free Speech Coalition. In 2012, the City of Los Angeles, the "capital" of pornography where 5% of all on-site adult film shoots take place, mandated that pornography actors wear condoms during filming. As a result, permit requests for adult filming dropped by 95%. Fearing the loss of millions of dollars in tax revenue, this condom mandate was overturned in 2016 (Lin 2012).

The COVID-19 pandemic negatively affected many industries. Entire entertainment industries, such as sports, theaters, and cinemas, were put on pause. However, online pornography sites flourished. According to Pornhub, compared with traffic on an average day in February 2020 (before quarantine), worldwide traffic to its site spiked 25% on March 25, 2020, when the company offered their premium service for free to incentivize quarantining at home and social distancing (Pornhub 2020). However, the pandemic did not only increase the consumption of online pornography; data also showed a 30% increase in daily private video uploads. This is especially impressive because the Free Speech Coalition called for a voluntary halting of adult entertainment filming by production companies in North America (in accordance with the government ordering nonessential businesses to shut down temporarily) during the early stages of COVID-19 (Dickson 2020). This is perhaps one example of the pornography industry influencing public health (and the economy).

More Than Just Pornography

Despite what some may think, there is more to internet sexuality than pornography. Where technological advancements in connectivity go, increased sexual activity will follow (or sometimes the opposite). An ever-growing list of sex-related online activities cater to every want, need, and fantasy.

As early as 1998, a "[m]ethod and device for interactive virtual control of sexual aids using digital computer networks" was patented. The patent described two computers, each connected to a webcam and a sexual stimulation device. Only in 2018 did this patent expire, allowing the field of "teledildonics" to advance exponentially. Teledildonics can be traced back to 1974, when Ted Nelson, a pioneer of information technology who coined the term *hypertext*, put a sexual spin on a device that turned sound into tactile stimulation (for reference, the internet was made public nearly two decades later in 1991). Today's technologies have merged human sexuality with the online world. Virtual reality (VR) and augmented reality (AR) technologies are perhaps the latest technology segments being shaped by the pornography industry (Trout 2018).

Advanced technology is optional. Technically, any form of online communication can be used as a medium for cybersex. Examples include searching for (online or offline) sexual partners or experiences, sending and receiving sexual messages, and participating in chats, discussions, forums, or comments sections on pornographic or sexual content. Once viewed as a sort of taboo, meeting partners online (on dating applications ["apps"] and websites) is now not only socially accepted but also the new norm. According to a 2017 survey, meeting online has overtaken meeting through friends for the first time (Rosenfeld et al. 2019). Whether looking for an erotic chat, a quick sexual encounter (a "hookup"), or a spouse, the Web has certainly made it easier.

Online Sexual Activity and Cybersex

The literature contains many definitions and categorizations when it comes to cybersex (Barrada et al. 2019; Cooper 1998; Cooper et al. 2004, 2000; Delmonico 1997; Wéry and Billieux 2017). Most researchers consider cybersex a subtype of *online sexual activity* (OSA), a general term defined as any online activity that involves sexuality with no specific purpose (i.e., entertainment, finding sexual partners, education, support, and purchasing sexual products and materials) (Barrada et al. 2019; Cooper et al. 2004). OSA has been categorized by some authors into three types (Shaughnessy et al. 2017):

1. Nonarousal, such as reading educational material
2. Solitary arousal, such as watching pornography
3. Partnered arousal, such as webcam sex

Others (Shaughnessy et al. 2011) have grouped OSA into

1. Informative
2. Relationship seeking
3. Sexually gratifying types

Cybersex has been defined as the act of consuming internet media in any sexually gratifying way (Cooper et al. 2004). Some researchers have further defined cybersex as sexual pleasure derived from online sexual talk (Barrada et al. 2019; Daneback et al. 2005). Cybersex may include watching pornography; reading erotic texts; participating in online sex chats, webcam sex, three-dimensional (3D) and VR sexual simulation or games; or searching for sexual partners (Barrada et al. 2019; Cooper et al. 2004; Wéry and Billieux 2017). Griffiths (2012) grouped online sexual behaviors as either cybersexual consumption or cybersexual interactions. For simplicity, in this chapter we use *cybersex* as an all-encompassing term referring to the consumption of any sex-related online activity, regardless of intent. We also use *cybersex addiction* when referring to excessive, problematic, or compulsive use of cybersex.

Addiction vs. Nonpathological Use

Why Is Cybersex So Popular?

The internet is everywhere, free (or low cost), and (for the most part) anonymous. This concept of availability, affordability, and anonymity is known as the "triple A engine" (Cooper 2013; Cooper et al. 2004). An almost infinite variety of cybersex content is available and can be accessed from anywhere at any time. This is especially true in the age of the smartphone and smartwatch. Sexual interests, desires, fantasies, and curiosities can be explored using an online alias, which can significantly reduce the risk of physical, mental, and social repercussions. Cybersexually transmitted infections are just computer viruses. There is less fear of rejection, especially for those with sexual interests or preferences that may be looked down upon by society. In this aspect, some users may view the internet as a safe space to explore their sexuality, potentially with the support of other people who have similar interests.

Four other "A"s have since been added to Cooper's original three (Cooper et al. 2003): acceptability, approximation, ambiguity, and accommodation (Hertlein and Stevenson 2010). *Acceptability* refers to the normalization of finding romantic partners online, which most likely extends to other forms of cybersex (King 1999). *Approximation* was first described in the context of men who were unsure of their sexual identity using the internet to approximate being gay through aliases and cybersex (Ross and Kauth 2013). However, this term can be applied to any use of cybersex that serves as a substitute or enhancer to real-world sex (Hertlein and Stevenson 2010). As technology advances, cybersex approximates offline sex.

Accommodation refers to the use of cybersex to explore one's "real self" (vs. the "ideal self") through sexual activities in which the person would not typically participate offline, such as partaking in riskier sexual activities that lead to infidelity by way of an online affair. Accommodation differs from approximation because it refers to the user's online versus offline *identities* as opposed to differences in the user's online versus offline *sexual activities* (Hertlein and Stevenson 2010). Finally, *ambiguity* refers to the difficulties in identifying what is problematic and what is normal (Hertlein and Stevenson 2010). This is especially true considering the evolution of social and cultural norms and variabilities among different groups. What one couple may consider normal, another may consider cheating.

Types of Users

There is no "one size fits all" description of cybersex use. Not all users have the same intentions, nor do they all suffer the same consequences. Although several researchers have proposed various categorizations of cybersex users, we discuss that proposed by Cooper et al. (1999a), who categorized cybersex use into three types: "recreational," "compulsive," and "at risk."

Recreational Use

Recreational (also referred to as *nonpathological*) cybersex use is what one may consider "normal" use. These users may wish to entertain or educate themselves. They have little to no trouble maintaining control of their use and are generally free of serious negative consequences. These users can limit their use, often lose interest with time, and may decrease and eventually discontinue their use (Cooper et al. 1999a).

> Jacklyn is a 19-year-old who recently moved to college. She is lonely and curious about the local dating scene. She downloads the most popular dating app used by the locals and begins to "swipe" Yes or No to other users' profiles. She "matches" with a few locals, exchanges messages with them, and goes on a few dates. This was entertaining for Jacklyn when she first started, but after a few weeks, she notices that she is no longer excited when she matches with someone. Her matches and dates start to feel repetitive and boring. As the semester goes on, she makes new friends and spends much of her free time studying. She spends less time on the app, eventually using it only sporadically, primarily on weekends and holidays. (Adapted from Cooper et al. 1999a)

Some recreational cybersex users may identify with the "kink" community, which celebrates nonconventional consensual sexual practices. They may connect with and find support from others with similar interests; buy, sell, or trade sexual apparatuses; or sometimes meet in person. Such online communities (often insulated and rarely visited by the general public) tend to normalize what an individual might have previously considered taboo.

Compulsive Use

The second group of users, referred to as *sexual compulsives*, are those most likely to have some sort of underlying maladaptive sexual preoccupation or dysfunctional sexual practice. They may have a past or present pattern of engaging in risky sexual behaviors or any of the paraphilic disorders listed in DSM-5 (American Psychiatric Association 2013; Cooper et al. 1999a).

Drawing from research on sex addiction, *sexual compulsivity* may be defined as an irresistible urge to perform a dysfunctional sexual act, associated with "denial, unsuccessful repeated efforts to discontinue the activity, excessive amounts of time dedicated to the activity, negative impact of the behavior on social, occupational, and recreational functioning; and repetition of the behavior despite adverse consequences" (Cooper et al. 1999a). Two large-scale studies (Cooper et al. 1999b, 2004) have shown that excessive time spent on cybersex seems to be an important factor in determining compulsivity because individuals in this group were associated with more negative consequences. For these individuals, the internet may magnify their underlying issues because it can serve as a safe space to explore potentially harmful interests without perceived consequences, such as social rejection, potential infection, physical danger, or legal issues (Cooper et al. 1999a). This is where the seven As described earlier, particularly accommodation, may play a major role (Hertlein and Stevenson 2010).

The consequences caused by their newfound behaviors can affect users and those around them. Some examples include infidelity resulting in loss of a relationship, financial losses from spending too much money on cybersex, or cybersex use resulting in a new substance use disorder. Other, more serious examples involve nonconsenting victims. This may be the case for those with certain sexual fantasies or paraphilic disorders, such as exhibitionism, voyeurism, pedophilia, bestiality, and frotteurism. Cybersex may provide a sense of validation for those with sexual compulsions or paraphilias (Cooper et al. 1999a).

> Jonathan is a 31-year-old single mechanic. Since receiving a pair of binoculars as a gift in his late teens, he has been fascinated with spying on his neighbors. What began as innocent curiosity grew into a voyeuristic interest and eventually into paraphilic disorder. He was recently caught and arrested after following clients to their homes and videotaping them in their bedrooms. As part of sentencing, he is mandated to seek therapy. After months of sessions, he reported that his interest in voyeurism started when he watched a pornographic video online with themes of voyeurism. He soon began only visiting voyeuristic pornography sites and eventually joined an online community for voyeurs. This community had a forum where other members would describe their endeavors and upload images and videos they had managed to capture.

At-Risk Use

At-risk cybersex users are those who may not have had any issues with their sexuality were it not for the internet. Despite lacking a history of sexual compulsivity, their cybersex use has caused difficulties in their lives. At-risk users can be further categorized into "stress reactive" and "depressive" subtypes.

Stress-reactive users are those who use cybersex as an escape, distraction, or coping mechanism when stressed. These individuals are typically socially well connected and have developed mature coping strategies when dealing with usual stressors. Their issues arise when facing hardships alone. They may rely on cybersex to provide a temporary feeling of social connection during stressful periods but may decrease their use (and revert to their typical coping mechanisms) between stressful periods.

> James is a 26-year-old graduate student who has been feeling guilty and lonely since ending his relationship with Stacey, his longtime girlfriend. To distract himself, James visits his "usual" pornography sites, as he has done since his teenage years (intermittently and without issue). One day, after clicking an advertisement, he decides to try live webcam sex with a model of his choice. During their session, James and the model converse, flirt, and eventually masturbate to each other. Eventually, James decides to reach out to Stacey. They date for another month, during which he does not think about cybersex. After another few weeks, Stacey ends the relationship, leav-

ing James devastated. Even worse, James has been feeling overwhelmed because his final exams are approaching. While studying on his laptop, he reminisces about his online sexual encounter and soon finds himself in another webcam sex session. Soon after, he develops a habit of engaging in webcam sex whenever he feels stressed or lonely. Although he wishes to stop this habit, he cannot and is too ashamed to seek help.

Depressive-type at-risk users are those who use cybersex to alleviate depression, dysthymia, or anxiety. Their cybersex use may be a way to feel emotions that they otherwise have difficulties accessing. These individuals most likely have a smaller social circle, spend less time with family members, and often feel lonely. For this group, sex can be a powerful way to alleviate depression or anxiety, and the internet delivers sex in immediate and unlimited doses. Cybersex use can become consistent with increased frequency over time for this group. They are less likely to become bored with cybersex as opposed to recreational users.

Josh is a 19-year-old single college student with a history of depression that he attributes to years of bullying in high school. He lives with his parents and mostly takes online courses. He describes himself as an introvert with few friends and considers himself a "loser," despite his success in school and as a competitive video game player. He first encountered online pornography when he accidentally clicked on a pop-up advertisement. After locking his bedroom door, he masturbated to the content he had discovered because it made him very excited. He went on to visit multiple pornography sites, almost daily. Eventually he found a website that hosted VR pornography and sexual video games that he was able to view with his VR headset. Shortly thereafter, he purchased a motorized silicone device that resembles a vulva in order to have the "full experience."

As his use became more habitual, Josh began neglecting his coursework and came close to failing a class. He tried to cut down on his use but was unable. He became more withdrawn, no longer playing video games with his friends. His depression worsened because he was no longer sleeping at night and had an intense feeling of guilt. After asking his physician for stimulants, Josh was referred to a psychiatrist who helped him with his underlying problems and his depression.

Definition

Despite research suggesting that cybersex use may have addictive qualities, no consensus exists as to its classification, pathophysiology, or diagnostic criteria. Even the terminology has not been agreed upon. Examples from the literature include internet/online pornography addiction, problematic cybersex use, problematic OSA use, compulsive cybersex use, and internet sex addiction (Chen and Jiang 2020; Wéry and Billieux 2017). Although most commonly classified as a behavioral addiction (currently, gambling

TABLE 2-1. Problematic cybersex

Uncontrolled and excessive use of online sexual activities associated with

1. A persistent desire or unsuccessful efforts to stop, reduce, or control cybersexual behaviors
2. Cognitive salience (persistent and intrusive cybersex-related thoughts and obsessions)
3. Use of cybersexual behavior for mood regulation purposes
4. Withdrawal (occurrence of negative mood states when cybersex is unavailable)
5. Tolerance (need for more hours of use or for new sexual content)
6. Negative consequences

Source.   Adapted from Wéry and Billieux (2017).

addiction is the only behavioral addiction listed in DSM-5), researchers have also classified cybersex addiction as an addiction disorder, a sexual disorder, an impulse-control disorder, and a symptom secondary to other psychiatric conditions (Hermand et al. 2020).

Wéry and Billieux (2017) found that among various proposed definitions for sex addiction and hypersexual disorder, loss of control, excessive time dedication, and continued use despite negative consequences were common criteria. In their review, they gave a general definition for problematic cybersex (Table 2–1). Table 2–2 uses the criteria for gaming disorder and applies it to cybersex addiction.

Cybersex vs. Pornography or Sex Addiction

Although quite similar, a subtle detail that sets cybersex addiction apart from general pornography or sex addiction is that some online activities have no offline equivalents. Webcam sex, VR sex, dating apps, and teledildonics all require an internet connection and cannot be done in real life (Wéry and Billieux 2017). This is not to say that cybersex addiction refers only to online activities that do not have offline equivalents.

Barry, a 24-year-old single gay construction worker with a history of dysthymia has recently been evicted from his apartment for repeatedly failing to pay rent on time. He has cut his work hours because he has been spending increasingly more time on dating apps. His routine involves swiping, matching, and sexting with other men on Scruff. He then stays up all night having webcam sex using a teledildonic device with other users he found on an online forum. He tells his therapist that he is neither a pornography addict nor

TABLE 2–2. Cybersex addiction (adapted from gaming disorder)

Persistent and recurrent use of the internet to engage in sexual activity, potentially with other users, leading to clinically significant impairment or distress as indicated by five (or more) of the following within a 12-month period:

1. Preoccupation with online sexual activity (OSA). (Individuals think about previous use of OSA or anticipate their next OSA. OSA becomes the dominant activity in daily life.)

2. Withdrawal symptoms when not engaging in OSA. (These symptoms may include negative mood states including feelings of sadness, anxiety, or loneliness.)

3. Development of tolerance—spending increasing amounts of time engaged in or searching for OSA.

4. Unsuccessful attempts to control the use of OSA.

5. Loss of interest or dysfunction in offline sexual behavior as a result of OSA.

6. Continued use of OSA despite knowledge of psychosocial problems.

7. Deceiving sexual partners, therapists, or others regarding the amount of OSA used.

8. Use of OSA to escape or relieve negative mood (e.g., feelings of guilt, sadness, loneliness, or stress).

9. Jeopardized or lost a significant relationship, job, or educational or career opportunity because of participation in OSA.

Source. Adapted from American Psychiatric Association (2013).

a sex addict and that he feels "free from his depressing and meaningless existence" when engaging in cybersex.

As in Barry's case, a critical element to cybersex addiction is "online dissociation," which was first identified in a study of excessive internet pornography users. It is defined as depersonalization and derealization (especially loss of time control) when engaging in cybersex for long periods of time (Wéry and Billieux 2017).

Diagnosis

Few screening tools are available for cybersex addiction, and of those, fewer are validated. Many have used scales intended for pornography, internet, or sex addiction, but these fall short in capturing addiction specifically to cybersex. Perhaps the most popular scale specific to cybersex is the Internet Sex Screening Test (ISST). The ISST was developed in 2003 and consists of 25 yes or no questions pertaining to five dimensions of cybersex addiction: compulsivity, social cybersex use, isolated cybersex use, money spent

TABLE 2–3. ICD-11 diagnostic criteria for compulsive sexual behavior disorder

A persistent pattern of failure to control intense, repetitive sexual impulses or urges manifested over an extended period of time (e.g., 6 months or more) resulting in

1. Repetitive sexual activities that become a central focus of the person's life to the point of neglecting health and personal care or other interests, activities, and responsibilities.

2. Numerous unsuccessful efforts to significantly reduce repetitive sexual behavior despite adverse consequences or deriving little or no satisfaction from it.

3. Marked distress* or significant impairment in personal, family, social, educational, occupational, or other important areas of functioning.

4. Exclusions: Paraphilic disorders.

*Distress that is entirely related to moral judgments and disapproval about sexual impulses, urges, or behaviors is not sufficient to meet this requirement.

on cybersex, and interest in online sexual behavior. Validation studies are only available for Spanish and Persian versions of the ISST (Chen and Jiang 2020; de Alarcón et al. 2019; Shalbafan et al. 2019; Wéry and Billieux 2017).

Although there are no ICD or DSM diagnoses specifically for cybersex, pornography, or sex addiction, options do exist. The 2016 version of the ICD-10-CM listed "excessive sexual drive" (F52.7) (World Health Organization 2016). The 2020 version does not include this diagnosis; instead it lists "other sexual dysfunction not due to a substance or known physiological condition" (F52.8) (World Health Organization 2020b). Inclusion criteria for this diagnosis are "excessive sexual drive," as well as the grossly outdated, heavily biased, and sexist terms *satyriasis* and *nymphomania*. DSM-5 also lists "other specified sexual dysfunction" (304.79), with its ICD-10-CM equivalent next to it in parentheses (Krueger 2016).

Recently, the World Health Organization (WHO) chose sides in the debate over the classification of sexual addictions. A new diagnosis, compulsive sexual behavior disorder (CSBD; 6C72), has been introduced as an impulse-control disorder (along with pyromania, kleptomania, and intermittent explosive disorder) in the upcoming ICD-11, set to be implemented in 2022 (Kraus et al. 2018; Krueger 2016). CSBD is defined as a "persistent pattern of failure to control intense, repetitive sexual impulses or urges resulting in repetitive sexual behaviour" (Kraus et al. 2018; World Health Organization 2019). Table 2–3 illustrates the full criteria for CSBD. As of today, this is perhaps the closest we have come to "official" diagnostic criteria for cybersex addiction.

Although certainly a step in the right direction, CSBD misses several important factors inherent to cybersex addiction. First, it makes no distinction between online and offline sexual activities. Second, given its classification as an impulse-control disorder, it makes no mention of tolerance or withdrawal. Last, it does not mention the role of emotional regulation (neither as a reason to use cybersex nor in terms of negative mood when discontinuing cybersex use, as in withdrawal) (World Health Organization 2020a).

Prevalence

Given the lack of common definitions or diagnostic criteria, it is almost impossible to know the prevalence of cybersex addiction. Several studies using online surveys have suggested a prevalence between 1% and 10%, with men using cybersex three to five times more frequently than women (Wéry and Billieux 2017).

Common Features

In their systematic review on online pornography addiction, de Alarcón et al. (2019) found the following predictive factors to be shared among different populations: "being a man, young age, religiousness, frequent Internet use, negative mood states, being prone to sexual boredom, and novelty seeking" (p. 91). In their study of more than 7,000 participants, Cooper et al. (2004) found that 11 hours a week was almost two standard deviations above the average amount of hours spent on cybersex. Their findings also confirmed data from previous research that the individuals who spent >11 hours weekly on cybersex were more likely to suffer negative consequences.

Common Associations, Manifestations, and Comorbidities

Table 2–4 is based on systematic reviews from Hermand et al. (2020), Wéry and Billieux (2017), and de Alarcón et al. (2019).

Positive Aspects

According to the WHO, sexual health is "a state of physical, emotional, mental and social well-being in relation to sexuality...which requires a positive and respectful approach to sexuality and sexual relationships, as well as the possibility of having pleasurable and safe sexual experiences, free of co-

TABLE 2–4. Associations, manifestations, and comorbidities

Class	Diagnosis/Symptom	Notes
Addictive behaviors	Internet addiction	Most common comorbidity
	Internet gaming	Associated with problematic pornography use
	Substance use	Very common; men more likely to use alcohol, and women more likely to use cocaine or benzodiazepines
Mood disorder	Major depressive	Strong correlation
Trauma related	PTSD and anxiety	History of sexual abuse in childhood very common, especially among women
Personality disorder	Borderline personality	Higher prevalence vs. population, as with other addictive disorders; insecure peer attachment (particularly avoidant attachment) and neuroticism also prevalent
Eating disorder	Compulsive overeating/ Bulimia; obesity	Very common, primarily among women; may be a mechanism to regulate feelings or because of body image issues with relation to viewing pornography
Online dissociation	Timelessness	Loss or distorted sense of time; most common type of dissociation
	Fantasy	Fantasy associated with cybersex
	Depersonalization	Objectification of oneself and others resulting in loss of self-identity; potentially a mechanism to resolve past traumas, as with PTSD
Sexual problems	Sexual dysfunctions	Associated with lower sexual satisfaction, decrease or loss of libido, and erectile dysfunction in males that is not present when watching pornography
	Paraphilias	More access to uncommon or paraphilic content online
	Hypersexuality/ Sex addiction; sexually transmitted infections	Cybersex addiction, whether stemming from or leading to offline sex addiction; sexually transmitted infections are common among this population.

ercion, discrimination and violence" (Greenberg et al. 2017, p. 539). Literature has shown that sexual health is a major contributor to overall quality of life (Greenberg et al. 2017). As such, cybersex may be a major contributor to sexual health and therefore to sexual and overall quality of life. As previously discussed, cybersex can be used to broaden one's sexual knowledge, inform oneself on a certain topic, or improve sexual or relational interactions or communications. Cybersex may serve to enhance one's existing sex life. For those unable to have live sex due to disability, sexual dysfunction, or any other circumstance, cybersex may be their only form of sex. Cybersex may be viewed as a safe space in which to explore interests and fantasies without social, economic, or physical consequence (Cooper et al. 2004).

Treatment

There are many unknowns in the world of cybersex and cybersex addiction. Much of the literature addresses sex, pornography, or other behavioral addictions. Empirical research on treatments specific to cybersex is scarce. With regard to sex addiction, several authors have suggested a multifaceted strategy that combines psychosocial, pharmacological, and psychotherapeutic modalities. In their systematic review, Wéry and Billieux (2017) found only three empirical studies that looked at treatment options for cybersex addiction. The first included 35 men with an average age of 44 years who attended 16 weekly group therapy sessions. Therapy modalities included psychoeducation, motivational interviewing, readiness to change training, and cognitive-behavioral therapy (CBT). The authors found that although quality of life and depressive symptoms had improved, cybersex use did not decrease. They speculated that this may have been in part due to the screening tool they used, because some participants did spend a smaller fraction of their time online using cybersex (Orzack et al. 2006; Wéry and Billieux 2017).

The second study, conducted by Twohig and Crosby (2010), included six men ages 21–39 who received eight 90-minute sessions of acceptance and commitment therapy (ACT). Five participants had significant reductions in cybersex use (online pornography viewing), with four of the five maintaining their reductions in use after 3 months. Participants were also noted to have an increase in quality of life and decrease in obsessive-compulsive-like symptoms (Sniewski et al. 2018; Twohig and Crosby 2010; Wéry and Billieux 2017).

Later, in 2016, the authors conducted the first randomized controlled trial in which they compared 12 sessions of individual ACT with a waitlist control in 28 adult males (average age 26 years) (Crosby and Twohig 2016). The ACT group had a 93% reduction in time spent on cybersex compared with 21% in the waitlist group. At 3-month follow-up, participants had an

86% reduction from pretreatment. More than half (54%) of all participants stopped viewing online pornography completely after treatment, and 35% after 3 months. There was no evidence that ACT improved quality of life (Twohig and Crosby 2010).

The third study, by Hardy et al. (2010), assessed 138 participants (97% men, average age 38 years) with problematic online pornography use and compulsive masturbation who were enrolled in an online psychoeducational program during which they received 10 sessions consisting of CBT elements and psychoeducation. Participants reported reductions in viewing online pornography, masturbation, obsessive sexual thoughts, denial, and negative affect and improvements in culpability, management of temptation/craving, positive affect, perceived self-control, and ability to be in a relationship (Hardy et al. 2010; Sniewski et al. 2018; Wéry and Billieux 2017).

Studies involving pharmacological treatments are few and are almost entirely case reports or case series. Thus far, studies involve the use of naltrexone or paroxetine (de Alarcón et al. 2019; Gola and Potenza 2016). There is little literature regarding the use of opioid receptor antagonists, antidepressants, or mood stabilizers for sex addiction and internet addiction (de Alarcón et al. 2019; Dhuffar and Griffiths 2015; Wéry and Billieux 2017). Naltrexone, an opioid receptor antagonist, has been approved for alcohol and opioid use disorder and has been used off-label in hypersexual disorder and other behavioral addictions (de Alarcón et al. 2019). Case studies have demonstrated reductions in pornography use with naltrexone (Dhuffar and Griffiths 2015). Antidepressants, specifically selective serotonin reuptake inhibitors (SSRIs), are known to decrease libido and can also treat comorbid mood, anxiety, and PTSD symptoms. Several case studies have examined SSRIs and various behavioral addictions, but results are mixed (de Alarcón et al. 2019; Dhuffar and Griffiths 2015).

KEY POINTS

- Cybersex addiction is conceptualized as a behavioral addiction, a sexual disorder, an impulse-control disorder, and a symptom secondary to another psychiatric condition.

- The triple A engine (accessibility, affordability, anonymity) characterizes cybersex and differentiates it from offline sex.

- There is no consensus and little research regarding terminology, diagnostic criteria, pathophysiology, epidemiology, risk factors, or treatment.

- ICD-11 includes compulsive sexual behavior disorder, which is the first "official" diagnosis related to cybersex addiction.

- Online pornography is the most popular type of cybersex.

Practice Questions

1. According to ICD-11, compulsive sexual behavior disorder (CSBD) is classified as which type of disorder?

   A. Addiction disorder
   B. Impulse-control disorder
   C. Anxiety disorder
   D. Paraphilic disorder

   Answer: B.

   The World Health Organization has included CSBD in ICD-11. As its name suggests, *compulsive* sexual behavior disorder is classified as an impulse-control disorder. There are no criteria involving withdrawal or tolerance, making choice A incorrect. As of now, paraphilic disorders (D) are the only exclusion criteria for CSBD. Although CSBD may be comorbid with anxiety, it is not classified as an anxiety disorder (C).

2. The triple A engine concept sets cybersex apart from offline sex. It postulates that the internet is affordable, accessible, and

   A. Anonymous
   B. Arousing
   C. Absurd
   D. Appealing
   E. Attractive

   Answer: A.

   The triple A engine model posits that the internet's accessibility (the internet is widely available and hosts an almost infinite amount of sexual content), affordability (for the most part, online sexual activities are free or low cost), and *anonymity* (users assume they are undetectable while online) contribute to the popularity of cybersex.

3. Morty is a 27-year-old single accountant with no significant past psychiatric history. He became exceptionally busy at work once tax season began and had also been worried about his cat, Tessa, who had been recently diagnosed with cancer. Morty was working extra shifts and long hours to pay the veterinary bills, for which he borrowed money. As a result, he felt lonely because he had not had time to see friends, family, or romantic interests. He began masturbating to online pornographic videos on his smartphone as soon as he got home in order to give himself a "break." Six months later, after tax season and despite beginning a new romantic relationship, Morty's ritual daily masturbation to online pornography not only persisted but had increased to mornings before work as well.

   Morty's online pornography use is best described as:

   A. Recreational
   B. Compulsive
   C. At-risk, depressed
   D. At-risk, stress reactive

Answer: D.

The passage mentions several stressors: Morty's busy work schedule, his sick cat, and his debt. He is also socially isolated and lonely. As a result, he resorts to masturbating to pornography to escape his stressors and substitute for human interaction. Recreational users (A) may have various reasons to use cybersex, but they often get tired or bored, and their use diminishes with time. Morty's history lacks any sexual compulsion, paraphilia, or dysfunctional sexual practice, making compulsive use (B) incorrect. The passage mentions that Morty's loneliness is secondary to his recent stressors, suggesting that he is usually a social person. Although stressed and probably sad that Tessa is sick, he masturbates to take a "break" from his stressors, not from an underlying depression, dysthymia, or anxiety (C).

Resources for Clinicians

Dawson GN, Warren DE: Evaluating and treating sexual addiction. Am Fam Physician 86(1):74–76, 2012

Zur Institute Online Course on Internet Addiction (www.zurinstitute.com/course/internet-addiction): Online course focused on how to assess and treat internet addiction.

References

American Psychiatric Association: Diagnostic and Statistical Manual of Mental Disorders, 5th Edition. Arlington, VA, American Psychiatric Association 2013

Barrada JR, Ruiz-Gómez P, Correa AB, Castro Á: Not all online sexual activities are the same. Front Psychol 10(February):339, 2019 30863340

Chen L, Jiang X: The Assessment of Problematic Internet Pornography Use: A Comparison of Three Scales with Mixed Methods. Int J Environ Res Public Health 17(2):488, 2020 31940928

Cooper A: Sexuality and the internet: surfing into the new millennium. Cyberpsychol Behav 1(2):187–193, 1998

Cooper A: Sex and the Internet: A Guide Book for Clinicians. Abingdon, UK, Routledge, 2013

Cooper A, Putnam DE, Planchon LA, Boies SC: Online sexual compulsivity: getting tangled in the net. Sex Addict Compulsivity 6(2):79–104, 1999a

Cooper A, Scherer C, Boies SC, Gordon B: Sexuality on the internet: from sexual exploration to pathological expression. Professional Psychology: Research and Practice 30:154–164, 1999b

Cooper A, Delmonico DL, Burg R: Cybersex users, abusers, and compulsives: new findings and implications. Sex Addict Compulsivity 7(1–2):5–29, 2000

Cooper A, Daneback K, Tikkanen R, Ross MW: Predicting the future of internet sex: online sexual activities, in Sweden. Sexual and Relationship Therapy 18(3):277–291, 2003

Cooper A, Delmonico DL, Griffin-Shelly E, Mathy RM: Online sexual activity: an examination of potentially problematic behaviors. Sex Addict Compulsivity 11(3):129–143, 2004

Crosby JM, Twohig MP: Acceptance and commitment therapy for problematic internet pornography use: a randomized trial. Behav Ther 47(3):355–366, 2016

Daneback K, Cooper A, Månsson SA: An Internet study of cybersex participants. Arch Sex Behav 34(3):321–328, 2005 15971014

de Alarcón R, de la Iglesia JI, Casado NM, Montejo AL: Online porn addiction: what we know and what we don't—a systematic review. J Clin Med 8(1):91, 2019 30650522

Delmonico DL: Cybersex: high tech sex addiction. Sex Addict Compulsivity 4(2):159–167, 1997

Dhuffar MK, Griffiths MD: A systematic review of online sex addiction and clinical treatments using CONSORT evaluation. Curr Addict Rep 2(2):163–174, 2015

Dickson EJ: Porn industry calls for shutdown due to coronavirus. Rolling Stone (blog), March 16, 2020. Available at: https://www.rollingstone.com/culture/culture-news/porn-covid-19-coronavirus-industry-shutdown-free-speech-coalition-moratorium-967788. Accessed May 1, 2020.

Glass J: 8 Ways porn influenced technology. Thrillist, February 14, 2014. Available at: https://www.thrillist.com/vice/how-porn-influenced-technology-8-ways-porn-influenced-tech-supercompressor-com. Accessed May 1, 2020.

Gola M, Potenza MN: Paroxetine treatment of problematic pornography use: a case series. J Behav Addict 5(3):529–532, 2016 27440474

Greenberg JM, Smith KP, Kim TY, et al: Sex and quality of life, in The Textbook of Clinical Sexual Medicine. Edited by Ishak WW. Cham, Switzerland, Springer, 2017

Griffiths MD: Internet sex addiction: a review of empirical research. Addict Res Theory 20(2):111–124, 2012

Hardy SA, Ruchty J, Hull TD, Hyde R: A preliminary study of an online psycho-educational program for hypersexuality. Sex Addict Compulsivity 17(4):247–269, 2010

Hermand M, Benyamina A, Donnadieu-Rigole H, et al: Addictive use of online sexual activities and its comorbidities: a systematic review. Curr Addict Rep 7:194–209, 2020

Hertlein KM, Stevenson A: The seven "As" contributing to internet-related intimacy problems: a literature review. Cyberpsychology (Brno) 4(1):1–8, 2010

King SA: Internet gambling and pornography: illustrative examples of the psychological consequences of communication anarchy. Cyberpsychol Behav 2(3):175–193, 1999 19178236

Kraus SW, Krueger RB, Briken P, et al: Compulsive sexual behaviour disorder in the ICD-11. World Psychiatry 17(1):109–110, 2018 29352554

Krueger RB: Diagnosis of hypersexual or compulsive sexual behavior can be made using ICD-10 and DSM-5 despite rejection of this diagnosis by the American Psychiatric Association. Addiction 111(12):2110–2111, 2016 27086656

Lin R-G: Porn industry may boogie out of L.A. over condom law. Los Angeles Times, February 21, 2012

Orzack MH, Voluse AC, Wolf D, Hennen J: An ongoing study of group treatment for men involved in problematic Internet-enabled sexual behavior. Cyberpsychol Behav 9(3):348–360, 2006 16780403

Pornhub: Coronavirus update—April 30. Pornhub Insights, April 20, 2020. Available at: https://www.pornhub.com/insights/coronavirus-update-april-30. Accessed May 1, 2020

Raustiala K, Sprigman CJ: The second digital disruption: streaming and the dawn of data-driven creativity. New York Univ Law Rev 94(August):68, 2018

Rosenfeld MJ, Thomas RJ, Hausen S: Disintermediating your friends: how online dating in the United States displaces other ways of meeting. Proc Natl Acad Sci USA 116(36):17753–17758, 2019 31431531

Ross MW, Kauth MR: Men who have sex with men, and the internet: emerging clinical issues and their management, in Sex and the Internet: A Guide Book for Clinicians. Edited by Cooper A. Abingdon, UK, Routledge, 2013, pp 47–69

Shalbafan M, Najarzadegan M, Soraya S, et al: Validity and reliability of the Persian version of Internet Sex Screening Test in Iranian medical students. Sex Addict Compulsivity 26(3–4):361–370, 2019

Shaughnessy K, Byers ES, Walsh L: Online sexual activity experience of heterosexual students: gender similarities and differences. Arch Sex Behav 40(2):419–427, 2011 20467798

Shaughnessy K, Fudge M, Byers ES: An exploration of prevalence, variety, and frequency data to quantify online sexual activity experience. Can J Hum Sex 26(1):60–75, 2017

Silver C: Pornhub 2019 year in review report: more porn, more often. Forbes, December 11, 2019

Sniewski L, Farvid P, Carter P: The assessment and treatment of adult heterosexual men with self-perceived problematic pornography use: a review. Addict Behav 77(February):217–224, 2018 29069616

Trout C: Teledildonics gave me the gift of long-distance sex with a stranger. Engadget, July 2, 2018. Available at: https://www.engadget.com/2018-07-02-flirt4free-teledildonics-long-distance-sex.html. Accessed May 1, 2020.

Twohig MP, Crosby JM: Acceptance and commitment therapy as a treatment for problematic internet pornography viewing. Behav Ther 41(3):285–295, 2010 20569778

Wéry A, Billieux J: Problematic cybersex: conceptualization, assessment, and treatment. Addict Behav 64(January):238–246, 2017 26646983

World Health Organization: Excessive sexual drive F52.7, in International Classification of Diseases, 10th Revision, Clinical Modification (2016 version). Geneva, World Health Organization, 2016. Available at: https://icd.who.int/browse10/2016/en#/F52.7. Accessed March 21, 2021.

World Health Organization: International Classification of Diseases and Related Health Problems, 11th Revision. Geneva, World Health Organization, 2019

World Health Organization: Compulsive sexual behavior disorder, in ICD-11 for Mortality and Morbidity Statistics, 2020a. Available at: https://icd.who.int/browse11/l-m/en#/http://id.who.int/icd/entity/1630268048. Accessed May 1, 2020.

World Health Organization: Other sexual dysfunction not due to a substance or known physiological condition F52.8, in International Classification of Diseases, 10th Revision, Clinical Modification (2020 version). Geneva, World Health Organization, 2020b. Available at: https://icd10cmtool.cdc.gov/?fy=FY2021&q=f52.8. Accessed March 21, 2021.

Internet Gambling

An Old Behavior in a New Age

Robert Rymowicz, D.O.

CHAPTER THREE

This was my first lesson about gambling: if you see somebody winning all the time, he isn't gambling, he's cheating.

Malcolm X

How can providers be sure that patients are abstaining from gambling, when access to countless online casinos is in their pocket? This chapter explores how gambling has changed given the rise of online casinos and gives providers the tools to address gambling addiction as online gambling becomes increasingly tempting.

Culture, Psychology, and Practice of Internet Gambling

Understanding Gambling

Internet gambling is quite simply defined as gambling over the internet, but to better appreciate the concept and the novel challenges this presents, it is first imperative to develop an understanding of gambling. Although DSM-5 (American Psychiatric Association 2013) defines *gambling* as risking something of value in the hope of obtaining something of greater value, it is widely accepted that such a wager must occur in the context of a game of chance to constitute gambling. In the United States, gambling is legal under federal law but is subject to significant legal restrictions at the state level, where complex and often contradictory definitions are created by both judicial and legislative branches of government. To complicate matters further, the term *gaming* is often used interchangeably, or alternately, to refer to gambling that is legally sanctioned.

A medically relevant definition of gambling is elusive. Slot machines, lotteries, bingo, and table games such as craps and roulette are widely accepted to be games of chance. Sports betting, and card games that favor skill, such as poker, should be understood in their cultural context as gambling, despite numerous legal definitions to the contrary. Reckless or impulsive stock trading could possibly be regarded as gambling and might share a similar pathophysiology. Games that allow players to risk something of value in a game of chance with no hope of winning something of value in return—an activity that is increasingly popular online but has no apparent correlates in the real world (see "Internet Gambling Beyond the Casino" section)—further befuddles any definition of gambling and invites us to consider whether problem gambling might best be understood as an irresistible attraction to the excitement of risking something of value.

Gambling Before the Internet

Gambling was common among all social classes in the United States in the 19th century. Progressive-era reforms geared toward eradication of gambling severely limited participation by respectable members of the middle class. The subsequent involvement of criminal organizations only fomented further opposition and made the legal repression of gambling a priority among law enforcement authorities. Moral opprobrium may have discouraged some vulnerable individuals from engaging in gambling, but legal restrictions in the 20th century ultimately severely limited access and availability.

Bingo halls and racetracks remained legal in a few cities throughout the 20th century, and lotteries grew in popularity after first being legalized in New Hampshire in 1964, but Nevada otherwise maintained a virtual monopoly on diverse legal gambling from 1931 until 1977, when New Jersey legalized gambling in Atlantic City. Gambling proliferated in the 1980s, with a rise in state lotteries and the passage of the Indian Gaming Regulatory Act by the federal government in 1988, which led to the establishment of hundreds of casinos on tribal lands. Glamorous resort casinos and aspirational marketing by state-run lotteries did much to rehabilitate the image of gambling by the 21st century, but access and availability remained limited, with many Americans living hours away from the closest facility.

Understanding Internet Gambling

Internet gambling first became available at online casinos in 1994 and grew rapidly in popularity as companies exploited the ability to offer access to users anywhere in the world, regardless of local laws, while basing their technical and financial operations in secure regulatory environments (Spectrum Gaming Group 2010). Attempts at legal regulation by opponents of gambling, who sought to limit or deny access, and by legal gambling entities, which sought to limit competition, led to the development of confusing and often contradictory laws by courts and legislatures at all levels of government.

Currently, at the beginning of the 2020s, online gambling is illegal in most of the United States. Some forms of sports betting are legal in 17 states, including Arkansas, Colorado, Delaware, Illinois, Indiana, Iowa, Mississippi, Montana, New Hampshire, New Mexico, New York, North Carolina, Oregon, Rhode Island, Tennessee, Virginia, and Washington. In 5 states— Michigan, Nevada, New Jersey, Pennsylvania, and West Virginia—sports betting and casino games are both legal (Play USA 2020). New Jersey offers more online casino gambling than any other state and falls just behind Nevada in total money wagered in online sports betting (Blasi 2019).

The New Jersey Gambling Experience

New Jersey has developed a sophisticated regulatory regime in which online casinos affiliated with licensed brick-and-mortar establishments in the state are permitted to provide online gambling to individuals over the age of 21 who access their websites or applications while physically located in New Jersey or by users with a New Jersey IP address. In practice, this has led to a rise in gambling tourism by New York residents to New Jersey train stations, where online gambling is heavily advertised. Despite minor hurdles in establishing an account, little is done afterward to ensure that the account is being used by the intended user, and a New Jersey IP address can easily be accessed from anywhere in the world by way of a virtual private network (Neal 2013). Although internet gambling at out-of-state or unlicensed online casinos is not permitted, the largely open nature of the internet means that legitimate casinos licensed elsewhere, unlicensed casinos, and fraudulent operations may be accessed with little difficulty.

All legal online casinos in New Jersey offer table games and slot machines, and most offer poker. Slot machines are the most widely played and most profitable form of gambling both in Atlantic City and online. Although the total combined revenue from table games, slot machines, and poker from all Atlantic City casinos is approximately five times greater than that generated by their online establishments, some individual brick-and-mortar casinos are less profitable than their online presence. Sports betting, which is managed by the same licensed establishments, generates close to four times more revenue online than it does at retail locations throughout the state (Division of Gaming Enforcement 2020).

Access and Vulnerability

Internet gambling presents unique challenges because of increased availability and access. It is available on desktop computers, mobile devices, web browsers, and phone applications. A wide variety of games, designed to appeal to a broad audience, are instantly available to gamblers and present few barriers to potential gratification. Access is available wherever the gambler has access to an internet-enabled mobile device and offers the opportunity for a high level of privacy. Patients often report engaging in gambling during times of stress and distress because they find internet gambling to be a readily accessible way to alter their mood. Individuals with gambling disorder often report that they find one or two types of gambling to be most problematic (Petry et al. 2006a). Female gamblers tend to be older and to gravitate toward slot machines and bingo, whereas younger and male gamblers tend to favor active pursuits such as sports betting and poker.

Online gambling may be particularly appealing to vulnerable individuals. Little can be done to stop children from gambling online, and problem gamblers, who may be excluded from gambling at retail establishments, may find online access easier. Pornographic gambling games, although not available in American casinos, are available online. Anxious individuals, as well as individuals who might otherwise attract attention, such as intellectually disabled persons or active substance users, may find access available online but otherwise restricted at brick-and-mortar casinos. Gambling disorder is often associated with poor health (Morasco and Petry 2006), and individuals with mobility issues may be more likely to engage in online gambling. With internet and mobile phone access now ubiquitous, online gambling is particularly accessible to people who otherwise could not afford to visit a brick-and-mortar casino.

Internet Gambling Beyond the Casino

Internet gaming disorder (IGD), as defined in DSM-5, specifically excludes gambling and games of a mostly sexual nature, but the distinction between video games and gambling has become increasingly unclear. Although competitive video games tend to focus on skill-based challenges, gambling-like elements are more frequently being incorporated into their ecosystems, with loot boxes presenting a clear example (see Chapter 1). The incorporation of gambling into video games may be of particular concern because gambling that begins during childhood is associated with an increased risk of developing gambling disorder (Burge et al. 2006).

Loot boxes have become a popular component of video games and consist generally of a virtual box containing an unknown virtual item that is only revealed when the box is opened and will often confer a particular physical appearance or some performative advantage to the player's avatar. The contents of loot boxes are sometimes exchangeable between players and may have an actual cash value. These boxes are sometimes given to players for free in exchange for meeting in-game goals, but they are often available to be purchased with actual money. Several nations have sought to regulate loot boxes; referring to them as "lottery tickets," China prohibits their sale to children under the age of 8 and limits their availability to those under the age of 18 (Hafer 2018).

Seattle-based Big Fish Casino further confuses any distinction between video games and gambling, despite appearing at first glance to be no different from any other internet gambling website. Big Fish offers gambling games that are free to play. However, it also permits players to add real money to their account to purchase in-game chips with which to gamble. Although chips may be won through play, using real money to buy chips allows a player to rapidly replenish an empty account, bet greater amounts, or take advantage of advertised special offers, such as chips being sold for less than the typical rate. Unlike traditional gambling, players may never redeem chips for cash or other real rewards—it is impossible to win anything of value. Multiple players, including one who lost $300,000 over 4 years, have sued Big Fish, accusing it of operating "illegal gambling games" and seeking to recover their losses through Washington's Recovery of Money Lost at Gambling Act.

Big Fish argued that their service is not gambling, by definition, because gambling consists of risking something of value in a game of chance in the hope of obtaining something of greater value, and Big Fish offers nothing of any value. The U.S. Court of Appeals for the Ninth Circuit ruled against Big Fish, reasoning that "if a user runs out of virtual chips and wants to continue playing…she must buy more chips to have 'the privilege of playing the game.'" This confusing definition would also seem to apply to any arcade game and has prompted bipartisan efforts to protect the state's video game industry with legislation to clarify that the Recovery of Money Lost at Gambling Act does not apply to money lost in games that do not provide a mechanism to withdraw winnings (Brody 2020).

With loot boxes and the decision in the Big Fish Casino case, regulators are increasingly willing to define gambling in the absence of rewards of actual value. If gambling might best be understood as an irresistible attraction to the excitement of risking something of value, then could it be possible to engage in gambling by merely watching another person gamble? If you have found slot machines to be less than exciting, you may be surprised to learn that at any given time, thousands—sometimes tens of thousands—of people are watching other people play online slots via live video streaming services such as Twitch and those provided on YouTube and Instagram. Some viewers simply watch, but others take a more active role, interacting with the player by recommending plays they feel might be lucky or by providing financial sponsorship.

Addiction vs. Nonpathological Use

Regardless of its legality, merely engaging in gambling does not constitute gambling disorder, and clinicians must distinguish nonpathological gambling from conditions that merit treatment. Gambling, particularly with regard to games of skill, may be an enjoyable pastime or even a lucrative profession. Individuals who engage in gambling in a rational and logical manner, approaching the circumstances with a well-reasoned understanding of the odds and an accurate estimation of their skill, might not meet criteria for gambling disorder. Strict application of diagnostic criteria may lead to unnecessary diagnoses among professional gamblers, who may be somewhat appropriately preoccupied with gambling.

It is not possible to determine the severity of a possible gambling problem based on the amount of money lost in play. A wealthy individual who engages in rated play at a brick-and-mortar casino may lose significant amounts of money, while collecting valuable "comps" such as free meals and hotel stays, without suffering any impairment. For others, gambling losses in the tens of dollars may mean having to sacrifice meals and medications. With gambling disorder, time may sometimes be a better indicator of severity than money, with some gamblers demonstrating substantial preoccupation and engagement despite no financial losses or modest wins. Compared with gambling at brick-and-mortar casinos, the accessibility and variety of internet gambling allows individuals to spend more of their day engaged in gambling.

The DSM-5 criteria for substance-based addictions require that clinicians identify use leading to clinical impairment or distress, as well as a minimum of two associated signs or symptoms, in order to establish a diagnosis. Although a diagnosis of gambling disorder also requires clinical impairment or distress, it mandates a minimum of four of nine associated signs or symptoms to prevent overdiagnosis. Fraud, criminal behavior, and other unethical attempts to gain money to gamble are rare among people engaged in non-pathological gambling. Those with gambling disorder are far more likely to experience relational conflicts and poor academic or job performance, or resort to absenteeism, as a result of their time spent or money lost at gambling.

Cognitive Distortions

Compared with nonpathological gambling behavior, problematic gambling is often associated with distortions in thinking, such as denial, overconfidence, a sense of power or control over chance events, and other superstitious beliefs. Online forums discussing internet gambling are replete with tips about which games are luckiest and conspiratorial theories about online casinos manipulating the odds to cause unexpected losses despite the most fortunate of circumstances.

Central to much of this is a belief in luck and some ability to divine it. Many gamblers engage in some deliberation before choosing a particular gaming machine or table, hoping to find something fortunate or familiar. Compared with their brick-and-mortar counterparts, online casinos have been particularly adept at offering a wide variety of cultural, holiday-themed, and specific interest-related appearance packages that generally do not alter the fundamental mechanics of the game but help promote feelings of luck and excitement. Despite being extremely popular, gambling games often feature appearances based on trademarked intellectual property, such as popular television shows or movies. These games often have worse odds for players to account for the licensing fees that the casino must pay to the trademark holder.

The concept of luck and other superstitious beliefs may be of particular significance in sports betting. Although sports betting clearly rewards skill, some problem gamblers report feeling compelled to make poorly reasoned bets in favor of supporting their preferred teams or players out of a sense of loyalty or a belief in predestination. The internet provides constant access to news that may affect the outcomes of sports matches and allows for constantly updating odds, fueling a cycle of researching and betting.

Individuals with gambling disorder may feel that money is both the cause and the solution to their problems. They may experience financial problems as a result of gambling that they then seek to correct through more gambling. This is often associated with lying to conceal the extent of one's gambling or losses and may cause a gambler to become dependent on others to provide a bailout. Gamblers may engage in "chasing losses," wherein they attempt to bet more in order to recover their losses. This is related to the "sunk cost fallacy," in which one overestimates the value of money already lost in an effort to rationalize further spending. The ability to link credit cards or bank accounts to online gambling accounts allows for play to be financed rapidly, with fewer opportunities for reflection and deliberation than might be possible in line at the cashier of a brick-and-mortar casino.

Escalation and Engagement

Online casinos typically allow far lower minimum bets than are permissible at brick-and-mortar establishments, allowing gamblers to play with small amounts of money and making losses seem inconsequential. Problem gamblers may find that they are not content with risking and possibly winning a few cents and may rapidly escalate their betting to achieve their desired level of excitement. Internet casinos often also permit higher maximum bets than are available at brick-and-mortar establishments or, if available, are confined to high-roller areas catering to affluent gamblers. Troublesome gambling may develop more quickly in internet gambling, which allows for a greater speed of play and allows gamblers to more easily play multiple games at once.

People with gambling problems often engage in gambling to alter their mood, which may then become dependent on the outcome of a bet. The availability of internet gambling affords on-demand access and is particularly easy to conceal from concerned friends and family members. Some gamblers report retreating to a restroom at home or work so they may gamble online surreptitiously and undisturbed. Individuals with gambling problems may experience withdrawal marked by restlessness and irritability when attempting to reduce or discontinue gambling and may find that internet gambling allows easier gratification than visiting a casino.

Diagnosis

Although DSM-5 qualifies that a diagnosis of gambling disorder should be made for individuals who exhibit symptoms over a 12-month period, it would likely not be prudent to withhold a diagnosis for individuals who exhibit severe symptoms over a shorter duration of time, given the increased preoccupation possible when constant access is available. Particular attention should be given to patients who feel compelled to conceal or lie about their gambling and especially to those who exhibit severe symptoms, such as jeopardizing relationships or career opportunities due to gambling or relying on others to provide money to cover gambling losses.

Individuals with gambling disorder who play online may not realize that they have a problem or may believe that their online gambling is somehow different from that of people who gamble at brick-and-mortar casinos. If gambling is suspected in a patient who presents with other complaints, the clinician should elicit additional information by asking how the patient spends money for entertainment purposes. Screening tools have been developed to distinguish normal gambling behavior from that which may be of clinical concern. Perhaps the simplest tool is the Lie/Bet Questionnaire, which consists of two questions derived from DSM-IV (American Psychiatric Association 1994) criteria that are thought to be the best predictors of pathological gambling. It asks, "Have you ever had to lie to people important to you about how much you gambled?" and "Have you ever felt the need to bet more and more money?" (Johnson et al. 1997). These questions are relevant to internet gambling, and an affirmative answer to either question merits further evaluation according to DSM-5 criteria for gambling disorder.

Positive Aspects of Using the Technology

Contrary to other uses of technology with addictive potential (e.g., internet gaming, texting, emailing, online shopping) that have obvious positive aspects, little good can come of internet gambling. Gambling disorder is often thought to be a solitary activity, especially when compared with IGD, which often involves collaborative play in multiplayer environments. Sports betting, which is significantly more popular online than offline, often features players gambling cooperatively and may foster closer social relationships. Gambling is a major source of tax revenue for jurisdictions that collect it.

Treatment

Treatment for internet gambling disorder is modeled on that for gambling disorder and consists of both psychosocial interventions and medications, although no psychopharmacological therapies have been approved by the FDA. A major obstacle to treatment is the fact that most individuals with the disorder do not seek treatment. This reluctance is attributed to several causes, including some of the cognitive distortions central to gambling disorder. Motivational interviewing has been promoted as an effective way to encourage willingness to change and is of particular value here because many individuals seek treatment only after having been coerced. Although abstinence from internet gambling is an achievable goal, improved self-control and reduced gambling losses may be considered practical successes and may constitute a viable harm reduction strategy.

Helplines

In the United States, the National Council on Problem Gambling maintains a free 24-hour, nationwide, confidential helpline at 1-800-522-4700 and an online peer support forum at www.gamtalk.org. Gamblers and their family members are encouraged to contact the council for information, support, and referral to treatment. Affiliates in 36 states, many branded as 1-800-GAMBLER, help coordinate treatment and often offer enhanced services at the local level, which may include free or discounted therapy or medical treatment. Helplines can manage acute crises, screen callers for gambling problems, and refer them to providers and to Gamblers Anonymous (National Council on Problem Gambling 2020).

Gamblers Anonymous

Gamblers Anonymous follows the 12-step self-help model created by Alcoholics Anonymous and is widely available, with free meetings in all 50 states and many foreign countries. Meetings are either "open" and accessible to health care providers and family members or "closed" and restricted only to people who desire to stop gambling. Gam-Anon, a sister organization based on Al-Anon, functions as a support group for families and friends. The 12-step approach is based on the belief that in order to recover, one must gain a sponsor, complete the steps, seek support from the peer group, and abstain completely from gambling (Gamblers Anonymous 2020). Gamblers Anonymous considers all gamblers to have the same disease and, as such, draws little distinction between casino machine gamblers, internet sports bettors, and video game gamblers, which may cause some gamblers to feel out of place. Limited data are available to support the efficacy of this approach for gambling disorder, let alone internet gambling disorder, but it is free and widely available.

Family Therapy

Family therapy is of particular value in the treatment of gambling disorder and is likely also valuable in the treatment of internet gambling disorder. Individuals with gambling problems are often reluctant to engage in treatment, and the participation of loved ones may be necessary for collateral information and to encourage adherence. Internet gambling may lead to significant relational discord and in many cases cannot be perpetuated without enablement through bailouts and other forms of financial support. Although evidence is limited, involving family in treatment is beneficial to address the consequences of internet gambling disorder and the circumstances that may perpetuate it (Fong 2005).

Psychotherapy

Among psychotherapeutic techniques, cognitive-behavioral therapy (CBT) appears to have the best evidence and support, with communities dedicated to improving this modality and numerous studies validating its efficacy in the treatment of gambling disorder. CBT is a flexible therapeutic approach that can easily be modified to make it more relevant to internet gambling and can be delivered both in individual and group settings. Although internet gambling disorder is somewhat similar to gambling disorder with regard to negative thoughts, cognitive distortions, and erroneous perceptions, a particular strength of CBT is its ability to identify the cognitive distortions unique to a particular individual. CBT for gambling disorder has been shown to reduce both the severity of gambling and the amount of money lost. It is an active therapy that requires engagement and homework and is typically conducted over 8–15 sessions. As such, it is most appropriate for motivated patients with at least some insight and an ability to sustain attention (Fong 2005).

Exclusion Lists

Some governments and casinos have established self-exclusion policies that allow gamblers to apply to be banned from gambling venues, with violators penalized by having their chips and winnings confiscated and possibly even by being arrested and charged with trespassing (Harper and Crowne 2010). Individuals are advised to reduce their access to cues that may trigger cravings for gambling. In practice, this could mean limiting access to gambling applications or websites by deleting installed software or activating parental controls to limit unsupervised internet access, closing gambling accounts, and unsubscribing from gambling-related email. In severe cases, abandoning a smartphone in favor of a simple analog cellular phone and restricting or canceling credit cards to reduce access to easily available electronic forms of payment may be reasonable.

Contingency Management

Growing evidence suggests that contingency management may be an effective approach for gambling disorder, and this likely holds true for internet gambling disorder. Studies have suggested that prize-based contingency management does not adversely impact gambling behavior among individuals with substance use disorders (Petry et al. 2006b). Less is known about its applicability for the treatment of internet gambling disorder. Compared with substance use disorders, which may involve substances detectable through laboratory testing, participation in contingency management programs to discourage gambling may be unduly reliant on honest reporting by participants.

Abstinence

Many gamblers may not envision abstinence as a goal and may instead seek to limit their play, pursue abstinence from some but not other gambling games, or restrict themselves from playing beyond a certain limit of lost cash. It is not clear to what extent such engagement continues to facilitate and perpetuate the neurocircuitry that underlies addiction. The extent to which individuals with internet gambling disorder are susceptible to IGD has not been established, especially with regard to engagement in gambling-like elements within video games. It is unclear to what extent individuals with internet gambling disorder should be advised to avoid any form of gambling, or gambling-like games in which no money is involved, and to what extent prolonged abstinence leads to improved self-control.

Financial Planning

A diagnosis of gambling disorder requires "clinically significant impairment or distress," which is not likely to manifest in a financially successful gambler. Because many of the psychosocial harms of internet gambling disorder are related to financial devastation, financial planning and advice may be indispensable to patients. Financial advice, which may include discussions of investment planning or bankruptcy, should be administered by competent authorities (Fong 2005).

Psychopharmacology

Psychopharmacological interventions are modeled on those for gambling disorder. Although no medications have been approved by the FDA, several have shown promise in clinical trials (Grant et al. 2014). Individuals with internet gambling disorder are likely to be similar to those with gambling disorder in experiencing high rates of comorbidity with other psychiatric disorders, such as mood disorder, bipolar disorder, generalized anxiety disorder, PTSD, and substance use disorders (Chou and Afifi 2011). Several studies have suggested a high rate of comorbidity with ADHD, which is suspected to be even higher among patients engaged in internet gambling or gambling in video games. The treatment of these comorbid conditions may be critical to the treatment of a patient's internet gambling behavior and should be managed in accordance with the best evidence-based practices.

Naltrexone

Opioid receptor antagonists should be considered first-line in the pharmacological treatment of internet gambling disorder (Grant et al. 2014), given their demonstrated successes in the treatment of gambling disorder. Numerous studies have demonstrated the efficacy of naltrexone in reducing the intensity of urges to gamble, gambling thoughts, and gambling behaviors, with individuals who show a higher intensity of gambling urges responding preferentially to treatment (Kim et al. 2001). Naltrexone appears to be effective in the treatment of comorbid alcohol use disorder and opioid use disorder and may show better results in the treatment of gamblers with a family history of alcohol use disorder (Grant et al. 2008). Studies have also demonstrated the effectiveness of treatment with nalmefene (Grant et al. 2010b), which is similar in structure and activity to naltrexone but has the advantage of lower liver toxicity, but this drug has not been commercially available in the United States since 2008.

Naltrexone is commercially available in the United States as an oral tablet, oral solution, and extended-release injectable suspension. Appropriate dosages for the treatment of gambling disorder have not been established, but trials have been conducted with as little as 25 mg/day and as much as 450 mg/day, administered orally (Victorri-Vigneau et al. 2018). Some studies suggested poor response at 50 mg/day, with several having escalated doses to >150 mg/day based on patient response. Naltrexone is subject to a black box warning that it has the capacity to cause hepatocellular injury in excessive doses and is contraindicated in acute hepatitis or hepatic failure (U.S. Food and Drug Administration 2013). Although no guidelines are available for the treatment of internet gambling disorder with naltrexone, it would be reasonable to begin treatment orally with 50 mg/day and escalate the dosage based on patient response. This may rise to as much as 200 mg/day, in a single dose or divided doses, bearing in mind the need to monitor for possible side effects, such as abdominal pain, restlessness, reduced appetite, and dysphoria.

Other Medications

Antidepressants were among the first medications used to treat gambling disorder, but controlled clinical trials have demonstrated mixed results with fluvoxamine and paroxetine (Grant et al. 2014) and no advantage over placebo with sertraline (Sáiz-Ruiz et al. 2005) or bupropion (Black et al. 2007). Limited evidence exists to support the use of mood stabilizers, particularly among gamblers with bipolar disorder (Berlin et al. 2013). Two studies have shown reductions in gambling behavior, cravings, and urges in patients treated with olanzapine (Fong et al. 2008). Evidence suggests that highly impulsive gamblers may benefit from treatment with stimulant medications, but caution is warranted because these medications may also precipitate gambling behaviors in individuals who rated low in terms of impulsivity prior to treatment (Zack and Poulos 2004). N-acetylcysteine (Grant et al. 2007) and memantine (Grant et al. 2010a) have shown promise in the treatment of gambling, presumably by reducing glutamatergic tone in the nucleus accumbens and thereby reducing reward-seeking behavior, and merit further study.

Special Considerations

Because internet gambling disorder is not an accepted DSM-5 diagnosis, individuals suspected of having internet gambling disorder should be evaluated for gambling disorder in accordance with DSM-5 criteria. Although internet gambling disorder may best be conceived of at this time as a variant of gambling disorder, distinctions between internet gambling and traditional gambling should not be lost on providers. Casino gambling in the United States has traditionally focused on table games, slot machines, and sports betting, with lotteries typically the purview of states. These forms of gambling are all available over the internet, but with an enhanced speed of play, permitting greater levels of gratification and potentially greater losses. Speed of play is of particular importance in internet gambling because of the phenomenon of chasing losses, wherein a gambler attempts to immediately recover lost funds. Internet gambling is far more accessible because it is available on any internet-enabled device and with a lower degree of supervision; whereas intoxication or overt mania might lead to scrutiny in a casino, these behaviors would be less likely to attract attention online.

Internet gambling also affords access to new methods of gambling that previously escaped the attention of clinicians. Gambling games in which players may risk cash without the ability to win anything of value, such as in the notorious case of Big Fish Casino, appear to have no equivalent in the world of brick-and-mortar casinos. The ability to watch gamblers live, interact with them, and send them money, living vicariously through them without engaging in actual gambling, is largely impossible in actual casinos but has drawn a significant following online. Gambling-like elements incorporated into video games in the form of loot boxes and paid services have transformed the world of video games and have blurred the distinction between internet gambling disorder and IGD.

As this distinction continues to erode, clinicians may find it expedient to diagnose patients with IGD as having gambling disorder for billing purposes, which may be diagnostically valid. Further research is needed to elaborate the similarities and distinctions between these two conditions. Individuals engaging in internet gambling disorder that is highly similar to IGD are likely to be younger and male, and their play is more likely to involve other people. These patients are more likely to be in school, and their performance there may suffer as a result of their preoccupation with gambling. Conversely, their engagement in internet gambling and video games may be critical to their identity and peer-group affiliation, and treatments and attempts at abstinence may lead not only to the loss of a stimulating activity but also to reduced social interaction and the termination of some relationships.

A key consideration in the treatment of both gambling disorder and internet gambling disorder is the matter of deception. Patients are often unwilling to seek treatment and may do so only after being coerced by concerned family members or employers or by the criminal justice system or out of desperation after substantial losses. Some individuals with internet gambling disorder may present for the treatment of depression or anxiety that is a direct result of losses sustained in gambling or the consequences of neglecting other obligations in favor of gambling. When internet gambling disorder is suspected, investigate further by asking how the patient prefers to spend money on entertainment and then administer the Lie/Bet Questionnaire. Individuals who endorse problematic gambling behavior may engage in deception by failing to disclose the full extent of their gambling, and their continued desire to engage in gambling may manifest as resistance to treatment.

KEY POINTS

- Internet gambling has forced clinicians to rethink some of the basic assumptions about gambling. Gambling may best be understood as an irresistible attraction to the excitement of risking something of value.

- The Big Fish Casino case and engaging in gambling as a spectator provide compelling examples of problematic gambling without any possibility of winning anything of value.

- The severity of internet gambling disorder is best determined by its consequences, which may be assessed in accordance with the DSM-5 criteria for gambling disorder. Although internet gambling may lead to substantial cash losses, many individuals may suffer more in terms of the loss of relationships and opportunities due to constant access to affordable play.

- Internet gambling disorder shares many similarities with internet gaming disorder, especially as internet gambling games become more like video games and video games begin to incorporate gambling-like elements into their ecosystems. Patients may fail to recognize that engagement in either may constitute gambling, owing to preconceived notions of gambling as being limited to traditional casino games.

- Patients are often reluctant to seek treatment for internet gambling disorder, may not recognize that it merits clinical attention, or may seek treatment for its consequences, which may manifest as low mood, guilt, or anxious distress.

- Clinicians may ask patients to describe how they spend their money on entertainment and should follow up as needed with the Lie/Bet Questionnaire, which asks, "Have you ever had to lie to people important to you about how much you gambled?" and "Have you ever felt the need to bet more and more money?"

- Treatment is available for internet gambling disorder. Patients and their families may find helplines such as 1-800-GAMBLER effective for managing acute crises and referring patients and family members to providers and treatments, which in some states are subsidized by gambling revenues and may be available at reduced cost or at no cost. Gamblers Anonymous is a free 12-step program similar to Alcoholics Anonymous, and Gam-Anon is available for free support for families and friends of gamblers.

- Evidence supports the use of cognitive-behavioral therapy in the treatment of gambling disorder in both individual and group settings, and although no medications have received FDA approval, evidence in support of the effectiveness of naltrexone monotherapy or as part of medication-assisted therapy continues to grow.

Practice Questions

1. Given that no medications are approved by the FDA for the treatment of internet gambling or gambling disorder, which medication should be considered first-line in the treatment of internet gambling disorder?

   A. Paroxetine
   B. Naltrexone
   C. Bupropion
   D. Olanzapine
   E. Naloxone

   Answer: B.

   Naltrexone should be considered first-line in the pharmacological treatment of internet gambling disorder given its demonstrated successes in the treatment of gambling disorder and a paucity of suitable alternatives. Several studies have demonstrated the efficacy of naltrexone in reducing the intensity of urges to gamble, gambling thoughts, and gambling behaviors, with patients who show a higher intensity of gambling urges responding preferentially to treatment. Paroxetine (A) and bupropion (C) have shown mixed results in studies. Olanzapine (D) has demonstrated some success and might be considered as an alternative in patients for whom naltrexone is contraindicated. Studies concerning the use of intranasal naloxone (E) for the treatment of gambling disorder are ongoing.

2. What is the most popular form of licensed internet gambling, in terms of money gambled?

   A. Poker
   B. Slots
   C. Sports betting
   D. Bingo
   E. Lottery

   Answer: C.

   Sports betting is the most popular form of licensed internet gambling in terms of money gambled, and online sports betting has eclipsed sports betting at brick-and-mortar venues in many states. In several states, sports betting has become more popular than traditional casino gambling. Sports betting is often not considered to be gambling, often not a priority of law enforcement, and widely available in states where it is not legally permitted. Sports betting includes fantasy sports, and beyond strictly sports betting, many websites are dedicated to gambling on the outcomes of future events, with presidential elections being exceptionally popular. Far less money is wagered in legal online poker (A), slots (B), and bingo (D). Although a substantial amount of money is gambled in lotteries (E), online lottery ticket sales are only permitted in 10 states and the District of Columbia as of March 2021.

3. Which of the following is absolutely necessary for a diagnosis of gambling disorder in a person who engages in persistent and recurrent gambling over the internet?

   A. Clinically significant impairment or distress
   B. Need to gamble with increasing amounts of money to achieve desired excitement
   C. Repeated unsuccessful efforts to control, reduce, or stop gambling
   D. Lies to conceal the extent of involvement in gambling
   E. Relying on others to provide money to relieve desperate financial situations caused by gambling

Answer: A.

Diagnosis of gambling disorder requires persistent or recurrent problematic gambling behavior leading to clinically significant impairment or distress, as indicated by the individual exhibiting at least four of nine criteria. Additionally, the behavior must not be better explained by a manic episode. Answers B, C, D, and E are among the nine criteria, but none is indispensable in establishing the diagnosis. Of note, the two mostly commonly reported criteria, which are not listed here, are being often preoccupied with gambling and chasing losses.

Resources for Clinicians, Patients, and Families

Gamblers Anonymous (GA; www.gamblersanonymous.org) and Gam-Anon (www.gam-anon.org): 12-step program similar to Alcoholics Anonymous and widely available, with frequent free meetings in all 50 states. Meetings are either "open" to health care providers and family members or "closed" and restricted to people who believe they have a gambling problem and want to stop. Gam-Anon, a sister organization based on Al-Anon, functions as a support group for families and friends. Both websites include calendars listing upcoming meetings with local contact information.

National Council on Problem Gambling (www.ncpgambling.org): Features a list of treatment options and contact information for each state. Council also maintains a free 24-hour nationwide confidential helpline at 1-800-522-4700 and an online peer support forum at www.gamtalk.org, which gamblers and their family members are encouraged to contact for information, support, and referral to treatment. Affiliates in 36 states, many branded as 1-800-GAMBLER, help coordinate treatment and often offer enhanced services at the local level, which may include free or discounted therapy or medical treatment. Helplines can manage acute crises, screen callers for gambling problems, and refer callers to treatment.

UCLA Gambling Studies Program (www.uclagamblingprogram.org): California residents may contact the program via the website or by calling 1-800-GAMBLER from a phone with a California area code. The program, in conjunction with California's Office of Problem Gambling, is available by phone, text, instant message, and email and offers a wide range of available services, including intensive outpatient and residential treatment at no cost to the patient.

References

American Psychiatric Association: Diagnostic and Statistical Manual of Mental Disorders, 4th Edition. Washington, DC, American Psychiatric Association, 1994

American Psychiatric Association: Diagnostic and Statistical Manual of Mental Disorders, 5th Edition. Arlington, VA, American Psychiatric Association, 2013

Berlin HA, Braun A, Simeon D, et al: A double-blind, placebo-controlled trial of topiramate for pathological gambling. World J Biol Psychiatry 14(2):121–128, 2013 21486110

Black DW, Arndt S, Coryell WH, et al: Bupropion in the treatment of pathological gambling: a randomized, double-blind, placebo-controlled, flexible-dose study. J Clin Psychopharmacol 27(2):143–150, 2007 17414236

Blasi W: New Jersey passes Nevada in sports gambling: should Las Vegas be worried? MarketWatch, November 9, 2019. Available at: https://www.marketwatch.com/story/new-jersey-passed-nevada-in-sports-betting-last-month-should-las-vegas-be-worried-2019-11-04. Accessed April 1, 2020.

Brody JM: Proposed Washington gambling law changes aimed at keeping state video gaming industry around. JD Supra, February 19, 2020. Available at: https://www.jdsupra.com/legalnews/proposed-washington-gambling-law-50692. Accessed April 1, 2020.

Burge AN, Pietrzak RH, Petry NM: Pre/Early adolescent onset of gambling and psychosocial problems in treatment-seeking pathological gamblers. J Gambl Stud 22(3):263–274, 2006 16816990

Chou KL, Afifi TO: Disordered (pathologic or problem) gambling and Axis I psychiatric disorders: results from the National Epidemiologic Survey on Alcohol and Related Conditions. Am J Epidemiol 173(11):1289–1297, 2011 21467151

Division of Gaming Enforcement: Financial and Statistical Information. Trenton, NJ, State of New Jersey Department of Law and Public Safety, 2020. Available at: https://www.nj.gov/oag/ge/financialandstatisticalinfo.html. Accessed May 22, 2020.

Fong TW: Types of psychotherapy for pathological gamblers. Psychiatry (Edgmont) 2(5):32–39, 2005 21152147

Fong T, Kalechstein A, Bernhard B, et al: A double-blind, placebo-controlled trial of olanzapine for the treatment of video poker pathological gamblers. Pharmacol Biochem Behav 89(3):298–303, 2008 18261787

Gamblers Anonymous: About us. GamblersAnonymous.org, 2020. Available at: http://www.gamblersanonymous.org/ga/node/1. Accessed May 1, 2020.

Grant JE, Kim SW, Odlaug BL: N-acetyl cysteine, a glutamate-modulating agent, in the treatment of pathological gambling: a pilot study. Biol Psychiatry 62(6):652–657, 2007 17445781

Grant JE, Kim SW, Hollander E, Potenza MN: Predicting response to opiate antagonists and placebo in the treatment of pathological gambling. Psychopharmacology (Berl) 200(4):521–527, 2008 18581096

Grant JE, Chamberlain SR, Odlaug BL, et al: Memantine shows promise in reducing gambling severity and cognitive inflexibility in pathological gambling: a pilot study. Psychopharmacology (Berl) 212(4):603–612, 2010a 20721537

Grant JE, Odlaug BL, Potenza MN, et al: Nalmefene in the treatment of pathological gambling: multicentre, double-blind, placebo-controlled study. Br J Psychiatry 197(4):330–331, 2010b 20884959

Grant JE, Odlaug BL, Schreiber LR: Pharmacological treatments in pathological gambling. Br J Clin Pharmacol 77(2):375–381, 2014 22979951

Hafer TJ: The legal status of loot boxes around the world, and what's next in the debate. PC Gamer, October 26, 2018. Available at: https://www.pcgamer.com/the-legal-status-of-loot-boxes-around-the-world-and-whats-next. Accessed April 1, 2020.

Harper M, Crowne E: Rewarding trespass and other enigmas: the strange world of self-exclusion and casino liability. Gaming Law Journal 1(1):99–121, 2010

Johnson EE, Hamer R, Nora RM, et al: The Lie/Bet Questionnaire for screening pathological gamblers. Psychol Rep 80(1):83–88, 1997 9122356

Kim SW, Grant JE, Adson DE, Shin YC: Double-blind naltrexone and placebo comparison study in the treatment of pathological gambling. Biol Psychiatry 49(11):914–921, 2001 11377409

Morasco BJ, Petry NM: Gambling problems and health functioning in individuals receiving disability. Disabil Rehabil 28(10):619–623, 2006 16690574

National Council on Problem Gambling: Programs and resources (website). Washington, DC, National Council on Problem Gambling, 2020. Available at: https://www.ncpgambling.org/programs-resources. Accessed May 1, 2020.

Neal M: Yes, people will hack into New Jersey to gamble online. Vice, November 26, 2013. Available at: https://www.vice.com/en_us/article/d73z8m/yes-people-will-hack-into-new-jersey-to-gamble-online. Accessed April 1, 2020.

Petry NM, Ammerman Y, Bohl J, et al: Cognitive-behavioral therapy for pathological gamblers. J Consult Clin Psychol 74(3):555–567, 2006a 16822112

Petry NM, Kolodner KB, Li R, et al: Prize-based contingency management does not increase gambling. Drug Alcohol Depend 83(3):269–273, 2006b 16377101

Play USA: Legal US Online Gambling Guide. PlayUSA.com, 2020. Available at: https://www.playusa.com/us. Accessed May 1, 2020.

Sáiz-Ruiz J, Blanco C, Ibáñez A, et al: Sertraline treatment of pathological gambling: a pilot study. J Clin Psychiatry 66(1):28–33, 2005 15669885

Spectrum Gaming Group: Internet Gambling Developments in International Jurisdictions: Insights for Indian Nations. Linwood, NJ, Spectrum Gaming Group, 2010

U.S. Food and Drug Administration: Vivitrol (naltrexone for extended-release injectable suspension) intramuscular. Full prescribing information. FDA.gov, 2013. https://www.accessdata.fda.gov/drugsatfda_docs/label/2013/018932s017lbl.pdf. Accessed May 1, 2020.

Victorri-Vigneau C, Spiers A, Caillet P, et al: Opioid antagonists for pharmacological treatment of gambling disorder: are they relevant? Curr Neuropharmacol 16(10):1418–1432, 2018 28721822

Zack M, Poulos CX: Amphetamine primes motivation to gamble and gambling-related semantic networks in problem gamblers. Neuropsychopharmacology 29(1):195–207, 2004 14571257

CHAPTER FOUR

Texting, Emailing, and Other Online Messaging

When Does a Communication Tool Become a Burden?

Heather Wurtz, M.D.
Donya Nazery, D.O.

What's not so great is that all this technology is destroying our social skills. Not only have we given up on writing letters to each other, we barely even talk to each other. People have become so accustomed to texting that they're actually startled when the phone rings. It's like we suddenly all have Batphones. If it rings, there must be danger. Now we answer, "What happened? Is someone tied up in the old sawmill?" "No, it's Becky. I just called to say hi." "Well, you scared me half to death. You can't just pick up the phone and try to talk to me like that. Don't the tips of your fingers work?"

> *Ellen DeGeneres*, Seriously…I'm Kidding

The best time to call me is Email.

> *Joe Chernov, Twitter*

Culture, Psychology, and Practice of Email, Texting, and Other Online Messaging

Written language and verbal communication make us unique as human beings. Significant advances in communication technologies within the past few decades have led to major changes in the way we send and receive information and connect with one other. The advent of email and other digital forms of communication such as instant messaging, texting, and social media have globally revolutionized how we exchange information, conduct business, and socialize. The undeniable benefits offered by these technologies have increased productivity and made life easier in many ways. Furthermore, the increased accessibility and mobile nature of smartphones have made these communication methods ubiquitous. Texting and emailing have become so ingrained in our daily lives that communication by phone, written letters, and even in-person meetings seem like a thing of the past.

We have become so accustomed to and reliant on these mediums that it is difficult to envision a world in which we function without them. The demands of modern life often blur the lines between work and home, and constant communication and availability have become expected as the norm. With the ever-growing personal and professional reliance on texting and emailing, as well as the societal expectation for people to be available at a moment's notice, it becomes imperative to discern when online communication crosses the line from necessity to addiction. This chapter examines how to identify and treat online messaging addiction.

Texting and emailing addiction, like other substance or behavioral addictions, refers to the inability to stop a problematic and compulsive behavior that results in significant impairments in functioning in various life domains, whether personal, social, or professional, over a prolonged period. It can lead to a decline in well-being and life satisfaction or to clinical depression and anxiety. Although it is necessary to refine ways to identify and treat more severe addictive patterns of texting and emailing, it is also worthwhile to pay attention to seemingly innocuous habitual use, which many people engage in every day.

Despite being the social norm, even the habitual use of texting and emailing is associated with significant physical and psychological risks. New research reveals that increased use of these communication methods on mobile devices contributes to distractions that lead to car accidents, interferes with exercise and promotes sedentary habits, decreases quality of sleep, and correlates with neck, shoulder, and wrist problems (Yu and Sussman 2020). Excessive use of texting and emailing has been linked to poor academic performance in youth and negative effects on mental health, such as anxiety and dissatisfaction with life (Lepp et al. 2014). However, negative consequences do not always mean an addiction exists. To identify a texting or emailing addiction clinically, functional impairment should be assessed by a mental health professional. One of the goals of this chapter is to help providers identify when online communication morphs from normal use to a bona fide addiction.

Previous considerations of texting and emailing addictions have mostly been in the context of the umbrella term "mobile phone" or "smartphone" addiction. Due to the novelty of these emerging behavioral addictions and the lack of existing consensus on terms, clear definitions, and robust longitudinal studies, recognition and accurate assessment of these technological addictions as independent entities have been limited (Yu and Sussman 2020). Although the concept of addiction has historically been viewed in terms of substances or illicit drugs, the new understanding of neurobiological and psychological mechanisms implicated in behavioral addictions has allowed for a broader definition. This is reflected in the inclusion of behavioral addictions, specifically gambling disorder, in DSM-5 (American Psychiatric Association 2013).

Nevertheless, some authors have argued against labeling these smartphone behaviors as addictions out of concern that the slippery slope of pathologizing common behaviors will generate a false epidemic (Panova and Carbonell 2018). These authors have argued that common behaviors conducted on the smartphone, such as internet shopping, social media networking, gaming, or viewing pornography, should be explored as their own entities because of the differing motivations, gratification, and sociocultural context that drives them (Panova and Carbonell 2018). Although these points are valid considerations, the 21st-century reality remains that digital communication is ubiquitous, with ever-increasing daily engagement with problematic and addictive patterns.

In 2019, global email users amounted to 3.9 billion people (Mohsin 2019). There are more than 5.035 billion text users worldwide, with projections for this number to increase over the next few years (Burke 2019). Even if only a small percentage of these populations meets specific criteria for texting or emailing addiction, these statistics suggest that millions of people may be affected worldwide. More importantly, special attention should be paid to younger populations, because current research strongly suggests that texting addiction disproportionately affects teenagers and young adults (Yu and Sussman 2020). Due to the novelty of these behavioral addictions, longitudinal and externally valid research studies are still needed to identify exactly how common and to what extent these patterns are present. The paucity of research and valid screening tools in this area should not imply that the problem does not exist but rather that we have yet to scratch the surface of the existing problem and potential effects of texting addiction on developing brains.

History of Electronic Communication: "You've Got Mail"

To have a better understanding of the current cultural context of email and texting addiction, let us review the history of how electronic communication methods rose to popularity, making their use nearly an obligatory part of modern living (Figure 4–1). It is hard to believe how rapidly these technologies evolved to dominate and consume our daily lives. The first electronic communication system began with what we now know as email. In 1971, American computer programmer Ray Tomlinson developed electronic mail and immortalized it with his signature @ sign. Soon after, email became a standard among academics, organizations, and dignitaries—with Queen Elizabeth being the first head of state to send an email in 1976. The growth in popularity of email paralleled that of the internet because it was one of the most useful and practical tools the World Wide Web had to offer at the time.

Email communication became more commercially popular in the 1990s as personal computers and the internet became widely available both at work and home. There were many benefits to using email for communication compared with the standard telephone; it was fast, efficient, cost effective, private, and had the advantage of built-in record keeping for easy reference. More importantly, email allowed for asynchrony between two people sending and receiving the information. Unlike a telephone call, both parties did not need to be present at the same time to communicate, and this allowed participants to control their schedules independently. The asynchrony in time zones was particularly useful for communication in the business world, helping facilitate global trade. By 1998, America Online (AOL), one of the first pioneers in email servicing in the United States, had imprinted the public consciousness with the famous notification phrase "You've got mail" to alert recipients that they have a new email waiting for their attention. Perhaps equally as unforgettable was the sound of the AOL dial-up tone, connecting millions of Americans to the internet so that they could browse the Web, check emails, and chat via instant messaging.

In the early 2000s, although email was mostly used for work, as it is to this day, instant messaging provided a medium for casual conversation and socializing. Instant messaging allowed for real-time transmission of written

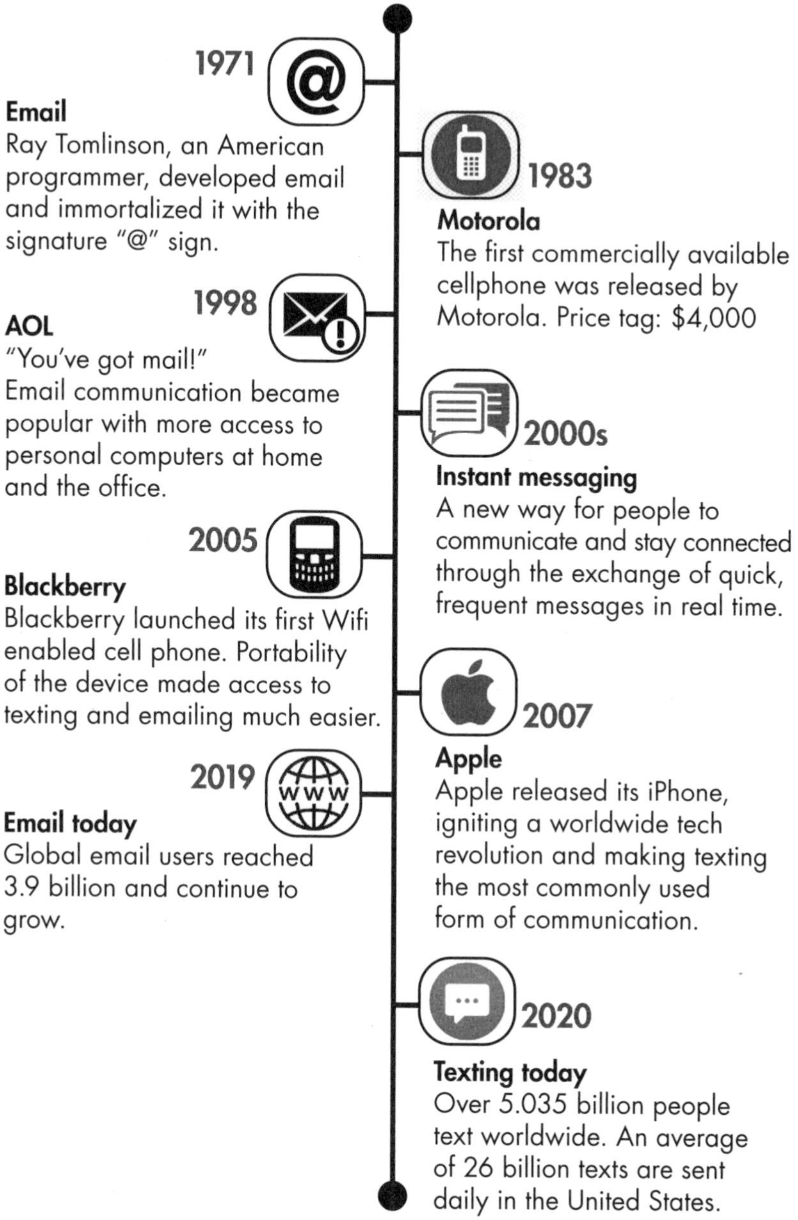

1971

Email
Ray Tomlinson, an American programmer, developed email and immortalized it with the signature "@" sign.

 1983

Motorola
The first commercially available cellphone was released by Motorola. Price tag: $4,000

1998

AOL
"You've got mail!"
Email communication became popular with more access to personal computers at home and the office.

 2000s

Instant messaging
A new way for people to communicate and stay connected through the exchange of quick, frequent messages in real time.

2005

Blackberry
Blackberry launched its first Wifi enabled cell phone. Portability of the device made access to texting and emailing much easier.

2007

Apple
Apple released its iPhone, igniting a worldwide tech revolution and making texting the most commonly used form of communication.

2019

Email today
Global email users reached 3.9 billion and continue to grow.

2020

Texting today
Over 5.035 billion people text worldwide. An average of 26 billion texts are sent daily in the United States.

FIGURE 4–1. Timeline of electronic communication.
Source. Data from Burke 2019 and Statista 2020.

messages between two or more parties over the internet. Unlike email, these messages were usually brief in nature and required the synchronous participation of users in a back-and-forth nature, mimicking real-life conversation. Furthermore, the messages composed were usually succinct and less formal in nature than email, making it an ideal mode of communication for personal, family, and social groups. Two important cultural shifts took place at that time. First, this was the first time in history in which technology blurred the lines between work and home life. Second, teenagers and young adults gravitated toward instant messaging for socializing because peer bonding is so central to human development during this stage. Instant messaging in many ways functioned as the precursor to texting, prior to the advent of mobile smartphones. It is not surprising, then, that text messaging continues to be the preferred method of communication among young people today for the same psychological reasons (Burke 2019). However, the exponentially greater access to electronic communication has created a greater potential for addictive behavior in recent years.

The rapid pace of technological evolution is astounding. We have come a long way just in the past 20 years, from waiting for our dial-up service to connect to the internet in the early 2000s to having instantaneous access to the "world" in the palms of our hands. Most people cannot remember the exact moment this transition took place, but the world has not been the same since. How exactly did a tool meant to help human beings communicate better become an extension of ourselves? Most people today are so attached to their smartphones that the device seems like an additional limb, difficult to function without and harder to part with.

Accessibility to electronic communication rapidly grew due to the portability of smartphones, their affordability (compared with the electronic communication devices of the 1980s), and the advent of wireless networking technologies such as Wi-Fi. The first commercial cellular phone was introduced by Motorola in 1983. It soon got the nickname "the brick" due to its massive size compared with today's standards. It also came with an impressive price tag of $4,000, making it affordable only to wealthy investment bankers and a few others. Almost a decade later, in 1992, the first text message was sent. By 1997, Nokia became the first mobile phone with a full keyboard, and by that time cellphones had become more affordable to the rest of the world. In 2005, Blackberry launched its first Wi-Fi-enabled cellphone. Just 2 years later, in 2007, Apple launched its iPhone, sparking a worldwide technological revolution that made texting the most-used form of communication, surpassing phone calls. In the late 2010s, mobile internet use exceeded desktop use.

In today's cultural context, accessibility to our phones is a double-edged sword. Although it has allowed for greater productivity, socialization, and entertainment, it has also brought the implicit obligation to always be available to answer messages as soon as they arrive. Many people may feel shackled to their phones by these social pressures and fear being perceived as rude if texts are not returned within an acceptable timeline. Similarly, employees may feel burdened with work emails even outside work hours. In this latter case, psychological pressure to constantly check emails and return correspondence may come from fear of not appearing professional in an increasingly more competitive work environment—even though studies have shown that checking emails less frequently reduces psychological stress and improves overall well-being (Kushlev and Dunn 2015). In addition to external psychological pressures, internal stressors also drive people to stay glued to their devices. An example of an internal barrier to digital "detox" is "FOMO," or "fear of missing out"—the anxiety one might feel when missing out on enjoyable group activities, such as being left out of a group chat (Przybylski et al. 2013).

Addiction vs. Nonpathological Use

When Does Messaging Become a Problem?

Today, many people use multiple forms of messaging throughout the day and depend on texts, emails, and instant messaging to communicate with both friends and colleagues. However, knowing when to stop is not always easy. Like other behavioral addictions, what is enjoyable, useful, or positive can become problematic when it starts to interfere with other aspects of a person's life. A clearly defined disorder for problematic texting and other messaging has not been established by the American Psychiatric Association (APA) at this time. Certain aspects of the criteria for gambling disorder, the only behavioral addiction to be included definitively in DSM-5 (and which is discussed in detail in Chapter 3), may be adapted to determine whether a person's use is problematic. Gambling disorder is included with substance use disorders in the "Substance-Related and Addictive Disorders" chapter of DSM-5 precisely because of the similarities between substance use disorders and behavioral addictions. We can apply these DSM-5 diagnostic criteria to other behavioral addictions, including problematic texting and messaging.

If use is problematic, the behavior has led to "impairment or distress." For example, people may find that time spent on messaging is causing them to decrease time or attention spent on other activities, including work, school, relationships, or hobbies. Their use may lead to a decline in career or academic performance or to limiting or discontinuation of other interests and relationships (American Psychiatric Association 2013). They may also experience symptoms common to other addictions. Withdrawal symptoms, such as irritability, anxiety, or cravings, can occur when users are removed from the behavior or device. They may be preoccupied with texting/messaging and have made unsuccessful attempts to decrease or stop the behavior. They may find themselves spending more and more time using the technology and may lie about the amount of texting or messaging in which they engage. In addition, they may use it when "feeling distressed" (American Psychiatric Association 2013).

Particular to messaging, people may find that they have "checking" behaviors in which they are often going back to their device to "check" for new messages or texts. This behavior can become excessive and impair concentration and functioning in other areas. This need for frequent checking can also cause people to experience distress and anxiety if they are separated from their device. The key question to ask in differentiating normal usage from problematic usage is whether overuse is leading to "clinically significant impairment or distress." Then, clinicians can turn their attention to additional symptoms described in the preceding paragraphs. In the diagnostic criteria for gambling disorder, four or more criteria are required over a 12-month period. Because there is no formalized texting/messaging disorder, the precise number of criteria is not defined. The more criteria that are met, and the more significant the impact on the patient's life, the more likely that the person has a problem with texting/messaging.

Assessing Problematic Use

Again, there is not a significant body of literature and research relating specifically to problematic messaging. However, using the similarities to substance use disorders and the behavioral addictions, specifically gambling disorder, one can extrapolate some questions that could easily be posed to patients during evaluation. Alternatively, the clinician could adapt a survey similar to the CAGE questionnaire, which is a short survey used to screen for alcohol use disorder. Most importantly, the clinician would want to establish that there had been some significant impairment or impact on function due to use of messaging.

Next, the clinician might examine whether the patient noted any issues of dependence or withdrawal symptoms, as described earlier. Does the person have cravings for the behavior? Does he or she feel irritable or anxious when unable to text/message? Of note, the amount of time spent on the activity can be correlated with problematic use but is not an adequate diagnostic criterion alone because many people spend a significant amount of time using messaging technology in their daily lives without it becoming a problematic behavior (Lu et al. 2014).

As far as actual instruments of measurement, Igarashi et al. (2008) developed a measure of dependence on texting entitled the Self-Perception of Text-Message Dependency Scale. This scale contains 56 items regarding text messaging and feelings related to messaging. It may be somewhat dated at this point due to the rapid evolution of messaging technologies; however, it can be adapted easily for use with patients today. A modified version of the original scale was recently validated with a U.S. sample of patients (Liese et al. 2019). Neither the original scale nor modified versions are in common clinical practice at this time but have been used for research and may be used in some form if problematic texting/messaging is suspected.

Addictive Properties of Online Messaging

Based on our current understanding of addiction, we can draw some inferences about what makes digital messaging addictive. For example, the instant nature of these communication methods can be thought of as quick onset or short half-life, which is also found in the pharmacokinetics of addictive substances. The instant gratification of receiving and sending messages strengthens our motivation and feeds into the impulse to continue checking our devices. Like other necessary and pleasurable activities, such as eating, sex, and successful social interactions, digital messaging works through our brain's reward pathways. In the evolutionary context, these are innate behaviors that ensure our survival; therefore, we are motivated to repeat them.

It is well known that dopamine is the main neurotransmitter released in the brain when one is engaged in pleasurable activities, such as socializing via text. When one is rewarded with a text, dopamine is released in the mesolimbic system, the brain's center responsible for pleasure, reward, and seeking behavior. This same center becomes dysregulated in addictions, making what was once useful and fun turn into a burdensome habit that is difficult to break. Other sensory stimuli, such as vibrations, sounds, and red icons, act as positive reinforcers to drive behavior through a well-accepted theory known as classical conditioning. The enticing "ping" sound of a text message, the tempting red notification icon, and the flashing email banner demand one's immediate attention, often interrupting real life conversations. The combination of classical conditioning and the dopamine loop make digital mediums addictive and hard to stay away from. Individuals with addiction repeatedly fail to control their behavior and continue to relapse despite significant negative consequences, such as poor academic performance, disrupted sleep, decreased life satisfaction, and strain in relationships. A new terminology known as "Phubbing" is used to refer to the phenomena of ignoring or snubbing real-life relationships due to preference for one's digital device or phone (Chotpitayasunondh and Douglas 2016).

Most Addictive Forms of Online Messaging

Instant messaging, texting, and other online messaging are more instantaneous and stimulating compared with emailing and therefore may be more addictive. The portability and versatility of texting increases access and the potential for addictive behavior. As mentioned earlier, text messages are usually shorter and less formal than emails, making them a practical, fast, and convenient mode of communication. The convenience of texting has recently made its way into traditionally email-dominated fields, such as business, health care, and governmental organizations. Younger generations tend to use email less often than do older people (Burke 2019). This decline is mostly due to the preference among younger people for communication via texting, instant messenger, and other similar social media applications ("apps") such as WhatsApp, Facebook messenger, Viber, Hike, and WeChat (Hou 2017). These popular forms of communication are more addictive among adolescents due to their instant nature and interactive interface associated with conditioned stimuli, such as red notification icons, sounds, and emojis.

The number of articles on text messaging addiction far outweighs that on emailing addiction. However, email use continues to be one of the largest modes of virtual communication to date and continues to evolve. Over the years, many forms of communication have emerged; however, email has continued to be preferred in business, academia, and personal use. In recent years, there has been a shift in the way email is used, with up to 60% of all emails now opened on mobile devices and 19% of email users checking their emails as soon as they arrive (Mohsin 2019).

Differentiating Between Technological Addictions vs. Using One All-Encompassing Term

Although the current literature uses broader terms, such as "smartphone addiction," this topic actually refers to the problematic use of content *on* the device rather than the device itself. Having consensus on terminology will help with the deeper analysis of the motivation and gratifications associated with each digital addiction and make room for the appropriate diagnosis and treatment. The most current literature suggests that distinct demographics are at risk for each type of digital addiction. In a recent review article, Yu and Sussman (2020) described that women tend to have a higher propensity to become addicted to social media, whereas men tend to become addicted to video games. Similarly, children and young adults are more affected by texting addiction than are other age groups. Some studies have suggested that youth with higher risk for digital communication addictions have shown more severe behavioral and emotional problems, lower self-esteem, and poorer quality of communication with their parents (Lee et al. 2016).

The smartphone is essentially a tool that allows for excessive use of its specific content, such as texting or emailing. It is important to differentiate which content is causing the problem. Social media, pornography, texting, emailing, and video gaming addictions affect different populations for different reasons. Identifying a specific addiction can help bring about greater understanding of the psychological factors driving the behavior and identify more appropriate and effective therapies.

Negative Aspects of Online Messaging

Sexting

Sexting is the use of online messaging to send sexually suggestive or explicit messages, which can include photographs. For mature adults, use of online messaging to send messages related to sex and intimacy may very well be an appropriate form of sexual expression. Sexting among younger people, however, is more complicated due to age of consent and level of sexual maturity. The motives for participating in sexting at a young age appear to vary based on gender. Young adolescent males appear to use sexting to build reputation within a male peer group, whereas young adolescent females largely participate to make a partner/intimate connection. Older adolescents, like adults, may use sexting in an intimate relationship as a way to connect with an intimate partner (Ševcíková 2016).

Regardless of user age, several problems are associated with sexting. First, online messages can be sent to recipients who may not expect or desire these communications. Because the content is often unknown until the message is opened, recipients may be exposed to inappropriate or sexually explicit messages that they do not wish to receive. In addition, because messages can be forwarded, the original message may be sent to other recipients without the original sender's consent. For example, numerous incidents have occurred, some involving minors, in which one member of a sexual partnership sends an explicit photograph that is then forwarded to a wider audience. Studies have shown that early, unwanted exposure to pornographic material can lead to negative results, including increased early promiscuity (Ševcíková 2016).

In fact, some of these messages may result in harassment if they are sent to someone who neither expects nor wants the message or if the messages are misused after a relationship ends. Furthermore, although online messages may seem temporary and ephemeral, they can be saved, either directly or as a screenshot, and then forwarded and distributed in ways not intended by the original sender. Young people now receive many lessons in school to remind them that once they "put it out there, it's out there" and to teach them that they should strongly consider the content of messages they send and anything they post on social media.

Cyberbullying

A study by Pew Research Center published in 2018 showed that 59% of U.S. teenagers have reported being a victim of cyberbullying (Anderson 2018). Along with social media sites and apps, texting and other messaging are the main platforms used in cyberbullying. There are several forms of cyberbullying, but many use online messaging. Some examples were discussed earlier, wherein an explicit message or image is forwarded to a wider audience than was intended by the sender or is sent to someone who did not agree to receive it. Other examples include name calling, physical threats, or spreading of rumors. In addition, a common form of cyberbullying involves harassing recipients by repeatedly asking them questions about where they are, what they are doing, and who they are with. Bullying is obviously not a new phenomenon, but using messaging and texting technology to bully is fairly novel and deserves attention by clinicians, particularly because cyberbullying has been linked to increased rates of suicide (Bailin et al. 2014).

Distraction

Online devices often lead to significant distraction from an activity the user is engaged in. Messaging can be particularly problematic in this regard due to the compulsive need to check for, read, and reply instantly to messages. In addition, users are most often notified that they have received a message with a sound designed to grab their attention. The detrimental effects of this compulsive need to instantly react to new messages have been seen in activities as simple as walking or as dangerous as driving. Many of us may have seen a video (https://youtu.be/bGpVpsaItpU), played for laughs, of a woman who is intently looking at her smartphone while walking in a shopping mall and then tumbles into a fountain. Walking while texting may result in a funny viral video, but texting while driving is so dangerous that national campaigns have been designed to educate and reform users not to read or respond to text messages while driving. In fact, as of March 2021, 48 states and the District of Columbia have made texting while driving illegal, and 21 states and the District of Columbia have banned cellphone use altogether while driving (Federal Communications Commission 2020).Texting while driving has been found to be a particular problem among young people and has become a major cause of death in healthy teens and young adults (Bailin et al. 2014).

Positive Aspects of Online Messaging

Text messaging, emailing, and other forms of messaging are important ways for people of all ages to communicate in the modern world. Currently, people in developed countries are using smartphones that allow them to be in constant contact with friends, families, and colleagues. Messaging is helpful to keep families who live distantly in contact. This chapter is being written during the COVID-19 pandemic, where stay-at-home orders are commonplace around the world. During this time of "social distancing," many people have noted the value of various forms of online messaging to stay in touch.

In reviewing the literature related to texting/messaging and addiction, most papers focus on the use of messaging technology to support patients. Messaging is used to remind patients of appointments, prompt them to take medications, and support sobriety. For the homeless population, cellphones and messaging have been life changing by providing a way for doctors, mental health care providers, and other community support providers to keep in touch with them, whereas in the past, a person without a permanent address was very difficult to reach.

In addition, some studies have suggested that the use of various forms of online messaging can serve as a way for people who are shy or have social phobia to interact with people and experience less stress. The composer of the message can take the time to frame, write, and edit the message without the pressure of facing the person with whom they are communicating. This practice can help people develop social skills that can translate to use in face-to-face interactions (Koutamanis et al. 2013).

Treatment

Psychosocial Treatments

Information and research regarding treatment of problematic online messaging is limited at this time and is, perhaps unavoidably, highly entangled with research on smartphone use in general. Logic—as well as some early research—would suggest that treatment of other behavioral addictions and even substance use disorders could be applied to problematic messaging. Psychotherapy, and cognitive-behavioral therapy more specifically, can help patients examine the positives and negatives of their technology use and make lifestyle changes that will decrease that use. Motivational interviewing can help patients explore their ambivalence about their use of technology, analyze their readiness for change, and evaluate the benefits they might reap if they were to "renegotiate" their time spent on messaging.

Mutual help groups offer some of the most important treatments for substance use disorders and behavioral addictions. Alcoholics Anonymous, Narcotics Anonymous, and more recently Gamblers Anonymous are central to the treatment of chronic addictions such as alcoholism, substance use, and gambling. They are commonly available in many communities, and extensive research has shown them to be safe and efficacious treatments. Although comparable 12-step programs are currently not available for texting or emailing addiction, it is interesting to note that support groups and rehabilitation programs are now emerging for the treatment of gaming disorders. Perhaps in the future support groups or rehabilitation programs will be available for messaging disorders as well.

Pharmacological Treatments

At this time, there is no evidence of effective pharmacological treatments for problematic messaging. As described, many researchers have theorized that behavioral addictions involve the reward circuits of the brain in a way similar to substance use disorders, and this theory is likely applicable to problematic messaging as well. In fact, one study showed that cellphone users found their cellphones more reinforcing than food (O'Donnell and Epstein 2019). In the future, research may examine whether pharmacological treatments targeting the reward circuit might be effective in treating texting/messaging addiction, like medications used for substance use disorders. For example, the opioid antagonist naltrexone, which has been used successfully in the treatment of opioid and alcohol use disorders, has been studied as a treatment for gambling disorder, with some positive results (Kraus et al. 2020). Although there is no evidence of effective pharmacological treatment of problematic texting, emailing, or messaging, such treatment is undoubtedly helpful to treat any comorbid psychiatric conditions. The treatment of depression, anxiety, and ADHD may improve maladaptive coping mechanisms that contribute to problematic messaging.

Special Considerations

Although texting and messaging are used most frequently by younger people and emailing is used more often by older generations, people of all ages communicate through electronic media on a massive scale. The related practice of "multitasking" has been shown to lead to decreased productivity, attention, efficiency, and creativity. Geriatricians report that, in the process of normal aging, multitasking becomes more difficult; therefore, older adults may find that attention to tasks is particularly challenging when messaging or emailing (Weksler and Weksler 2012). As a result, clinicians should make sure to evaluate and discuss the possibility of texting/messaging addiction in people of all ages, specifically not neglecting the older patient population.

Email has become a major arena for criminal scams and identity theft. For example, hackers send emails that appear to be from family members, friends, or the person's bank and either ask recipients to fill in user data, including personal information and passwords, or ask them to sign up for various scams. Unfortunately, elderly users are disproportionately affected. Although young people do also fall prey to email scams, hacks, and "phishing," they have grown up "side-by-side" with such malevolent technologies and appear to be somewhat more savvy when it comes to discerning criminal activity in their email inbox. It is helpful to people of all ages, but particularly older people who may be particularly vulnerable to "phishing" scams and other electronic crimes, to be educated on how to recognize texting and emailing scams.

KEY POINTS

- Since the advent of email in the 1970s, technological communication has grown and evolved significantly. Today, text messaging is one of the most common methods of communication, with messaging applications gaining recent popularity.

- Online messaging has become a vital part of modern-day communication, both personally and professionally.

- Despite the unquestionable utility of online messaging, the instant availability and demand for rapid response sometimes leads to problematic use or addiction that severely interferes with a person's life.

- Young people are the predominant users of various messaging technologies, but people of all ages can be at risk for problematic use.

- For screening, diagnosis, and treatment of problematic messaging, substance use disorders and behavioral addictions can serve as a road map because specific research is limited at this time.

Practice Questions

1. Which of the following would be most likely to indicate that a patient's texting has become problematic?

   A. Texting is the patient's primary means of communication.
   B. Texting has led to significant impairment or distress.
   C. A significant amount of time is spent daily on texting.
   D. The patient responds eagerly and quickly to notifications of new texts.
   E. The patient sends texts to other people while at gatherings or meetings.

   Answer: B.

   Extrapolating from the diagnostic criteria for gambling disorder, in order to diagnose problematic texting, evidence must indicate significant impairment or distress, including effects on career, school, or relationships; withdrawal symptoms when removed from the activity; and other criteria as discussed. Texting is a common communication method, particularly among young people, who use it as a primary means of communication, thus option A would not necessarily be problematic. Many people spend a significant amount of time on texting each day, but if it is not leading to any impairment, option C is not indicative of problematic behavior. "Checking" behavior that interferes with other activities could become problematic, but eager and quick response to text messages (D) is not in itself a problem. Although it may be rude or insensitive to send texts while at a gathering or meeting (E), unless it leads to problems in job performance or relationships, it does not indicate texting addiction.

2. Of the following choices, which would be the first-line pharmaceutical treatment for a patient with major depressive disorder who appears to show signs of addiction to email?

   A. Naltrexone
   B. Aripiprazole
   C. Varenicline
   D. Fluoxetine
   E. Lithium

   Answer: D.

Although no significant evidence is yet available for the use of medications to treat addiction to email, clinicians should certainly treat any underlying or comorbid psychiatric conditions. For this patient with major depressive disorder, a selective serotonin reuptake inhibitor, such as fluoxetine, would be a good first-line treatment option. Naltrexone (A) has been used for alcohol and opioid use disorders and has shown some positive results in gambling disorder. However, it has not been studied in email addiction, and no evidence currently supports its use. Aripiprazole (B) is a second-generation antipsychotic medication used for psychotic disorders, bipolar disorder, and as an augmentation strategy in depressive disorders, but it would not be a first-line treatment for this patient. Varenicline (C) is a medication used for smoking cessation, and lithium (E) is used to treat bipolar disorder; neither would be indicated in this case.

3. There are several similarities between substance use disorders and behavioral addictions, specifically gambling disorder. Which of the following symptoms is specific to problematic texting/messaging?

    A. Use when feeling distressed
    B. Withdrawal symptoms such as cravings, irritability, and anxiety
    C. "Checking" behaviors
    D. Lying about frequency of use
    E. Damage to relationships, career, or hobbies

    Answer: C.

    The need to keep checking for new messages is specific to problematic texting/messaging, may decrease users' ability to concentrate, and can lead to anxiety when they are separated from their devices. The other choices (A, B, D, E) are common to substance use disorders and gambling disorder, as well as to problematic texting/messaging.

Resources for Clinicians, Patients, and Families

American Psychological Association (www.apa.org)
Motivational Interviewing Network of Trainers (MINT; www.motivationalinterviewing.org): An international resource for training in motivational interviewing.

Psychology Today (www.psychologytoday.com): A good resource for patients, with down-to-earth articles on many subjects that offer several different ways to look at behavior and many suggestions for making changes. Site is an easily searchable and free online resource.

Screen/Life Balance (www.screenlifebalance.com): This website, by Catherine Price, author of the book, *How to Break Up With Your Phone: The 30-Day Plan to Take Back Your Life*, provides practical tips on minimizing screen time.

References

American Psychiatric Association: Diagnostic and Statistical Manual of Mental Disorders, 5th Edition. Arlington, VA, American Psychiatric Association, 2013

Anderson M: A majority of teens have experienced some form of cyberbullying. Pew Research Center, 2018. Available at: http://search.proquest.com/docview/2127647261/?pq-origsite=primo. Accessed May 11, 2020.

Bailin A, Milanaik R, Adesman A: Health implications of new age technologies for adolescents: a review of the research. Curr Opin Pediatr 26(5):605–619, 2014 25160783

Burke K: 107 Texting statistics that answer all your questions. Textrequest.com, 2019. Available at: https://www.textrequest.com/blog/texting-statistics-answer-questions. Accessed May 17, 2020.

Chotpitayasunondh V, Douglas KM: How "phubbing" becomes the norm: the antecedents and consequences of snubbing via smartphone. Comput Human Behav 63:9–18, 2016

Federal Communications Commission: The dangers of distracted driving. FCC.com, 2020. Available at: https://www.fcc.gov/consumers/guides/dangers-texting-while-driving. Accessed March 22, 2021.

Hou S: Measuring social media active level (SMACTIVE) and engagement level (SMENGAGE) among professionals in higher education. International Journal of Cyber Society and Education 10(1):1–16, 2017

Igarashi T, Motoyoshi T, Takai J, Yoshida T: No mobile, no life: self-perception and text-message dependency among Japanese high school students. Comput Human Behav 24(5):2311–2324, 2008

Koutamanis M, Vossen HGM, Peter J, Valkenburg PM: Practice makes perfect: the longitudinal effect of adolescents' instant messaging on their ability to initiate offline friendships. Comput Human Behav 29(6):2265–2272, 2013

Kraus SW, Etuk R, Potenza MN: Current pharmacotherapy for gambling disorder: a systematic review. Expert Opin Pharmacother 21(3):287–296, 2020 31928246

Kushlev K, Dunn EW: Checking email less frequently reduces stress. Comput Human Behav 43(February):220–228, 2015

Lee J, Sung M, Song S, et al: Psychological factors associated with smartphone addiction in South Korean adolescents. J Early Adolesc 38(3):288–302, 2016

Lepp A, Barkley JE, Karpinski AC: The relationship between cell phone use, academic performance, anxiety, and satisfaction with life in college students. Comput Human Behav 31(February):343–350, 2014

Liese BS, Benau EM, Atchley P, et al: The Self-perception of Text-message Dependency Scale (STDS): psychometric update based on a United States sample. Am J Drug Alcohol Abuse 45(1):42–50, 2019 29757688

Lu X, Katoh T, Chen Z, et al: Text messaging: are dependency and excessive use discretely different for Japanese university students? Psychiatry Res 216(2):255–262, 2014 24560613

Mohsin M: 10 Email marketing stats you need to know in 2020. Oberlo.com, 2019. Available at: https://www.oberlo.com/blog/email-marketing-statistics. Accessed May 11, 2020.

O'Donnell S, Epstein LH: Smartphones are more reinforcing than food for students. Addict Behav 90:124–133, 2019 30390436

Panova T, Carbonell X: Is smartphone addiction really an addiction? J Behav Addict 7(2):252–259, 2018 29895183

Przybylski AK, Murayama K, DeHaan CR, Gladwell V: Motivational, emotional, and behavioral correlates of fear of missing out. Comput Human Behav 29(4):1841–1848, 2013

Ševčíková A: Girls' and boys' experience with teen sexting in early and late adolescence. J Adolesc 51:156–162, 2016 27391169

Statisa: Number of e-mail users worldwide from 2017 to 2025 (in millions). Statista.com, 2020. Available at: https://www.statista.com/statistics/255080/number-of-e-mail-users-worldwide. Accessed May 17, 2020.

Weksler ME, Weksler BB: The epidemic of distraction. Gerontology 58(5):385–390, 2012 22572729

Yu S, Sussman S: Does smartphone addiction fall on a continuum of addictive behaviors? Int J Environ Res Public Health 17(2):422, 2020 31936316

Internet Surfing and Information Overload

Diego Garces Grosse, M.D.

Don't slide down the rabbit hole. The way down is a breeze, but climbing back's a battle.

Kate Morton, The Clockmaker's Daughter

Culture, Psychology, and Practice of Internet Addiction

The World Wide Web

The groundwork for what would eventually become the internet was laid down at the European Organization for Nuclear Research in 1989. British engineer and computer scientist Tim Berners-Lee wanted to develop a system that would allow physicists to share information in a virtual database where it would not be lost. In 1989, Berners-Lee proposed the creation of "a large hypertext database with typed links" (p. 11) and described his concept as "a way to link and access information of various kinds as a web of nodes in which the user can browse at will" providing access to "many large classes of stored information such as reports, notes, data-bases, computer documentation and on-line systems" (Berners-Lee and Cailliau 1990, p. 1). What Berners-Lee initially created for sharing information between scientists around the world became widespread quickly, and by 1991 the World Wide Web was available in several countries. It was indeed a large database of technical documents that scientists could browse freely, with links between documents.

By 1993, the internet was opened to the public, which triggered the creation of browsers and servers. Information of all kinds flooded the World Wide Web, and hypertexts were used as the paths linking content. These hypertexts, also known as links, would soon create what rapidly became known as Web surfing. Unceasing advancements in technology have led to wider internet availability around the world, with an ever-growing number of users. By 1995, roughly 1% of the world population had access to the internet, and by 2016, that number had grown to 46%. Growth continues rapidly to this day; in 2020, roughly 57% of the world population had access to the internet, with more than 4.5 billion users a day (Statista 2020).

Internet Surfing

Internet surfing refers to the practice of jumping from one Web page to another via hyperlinks. This surfing is usually done in an undirected manner, typically by following the momentary interest or attention of the user. The internet is a space in which information can be easily shared, and the body of information continues to grow every day. This makes it an amazing source of information with one major caveat: When looking for something specific, the user may become sidetracked, finding a plethora of related information that can complement the topic being explored. In many cases, this additional information can be beneficial, but many times information can veer off topic. Internet searches may quickly propel the user into vague internet surfing without a clear objective, particularly on websites in which clicking on a word will open a new topic.

Sites for open discussion, such as Reddit, and wikis, such as Wikipedia, enable users to surf the Web to an unlimited extent. Reddit allows the user to follow threads of discussion that often have links to discussions of similar topics, therefore creating a never-ending journey from one discussion to another. Wikipedia, in a similar manner, offers articles that usually present precise and concise information and have embedded links to other articles on other topics, some of which are unrelated or barely mentioned in the initial article. Both websites have seen a major increase in users and content over time. Reddit users have increased 30%, from 330 million in 2018 to 430 million in 2019. Reddit posts increased from 153 million in 2018 to 199 million in 2019 (Foundation Inc. 2019). Wikipedia has seen astounding growth, from about 200,000 articles in 2002 to more than 52 million in 309 languages, and nearing 40 million users, by March 2021 (Wikipedia 2021).

Wikipedia's article on "Internet" (https://en.wikipedia.org/wiki/Internet) is a fascinating example of information overload. Every paragraph in the article has highlighted words—hypertext links—that take the user to a different article. For example, if the user clicks on the word "academia," they are taken to the article "Academy," which has its own hypertext links to many more different articles. If this process of clicking hypertexts continues, what began as a search on the topic of the internet can end up in an article about ancient Greek warfare.

This is an example of what would be considered internet surfing—going from one Web page to another without a clear path or objective. Going a little further, Wikipedia has more than 6 million articles in English and more than 52 million in 309 languages (Wikipedia 2021), most of which are interconnected by a seemingly infinite network of hypertext links. This high level of interconnection led users to develop a game in which they challenge each other to go from a random starting Wikipedia article to an unrelated article in the fewest steps possible.

Due to advancements in technology, surfing the Web now encompasses reading articles and watching countless videos and requires less effort from the user. YouTube and Vimeo allow internet surfers to access multitudes of information by watching or listening, with related videos being advertised constantly—an evolution of the hyperlink chain. The autoplay feature on these sites adds to the complexity because videos will keep rolling, one after another, if the user does not stop them. Internet surfing has become a multimedia buffet and is no longer confined to the written word. If not properly directed, Web surfing can quickly become hours of nonproductive browsing, to the point at which the surfer may "drown" in information.

Addiction vs. Nonpathological Use

How Can We Define Internet Addiction?

Internet gaming disorder (IGD; see Chapter 1) has been highlighted in Section III of DSM-5 (American Psychiatric Association 2013) as a condition requiring further study. However, IGD excludes other problematic behaviors related to internet use, such as gambling or excessive social media use. Internet addiction (IA) by itself is not recognized as a diagnosis. Because of this, there is no consensus on how to define IA or which criteria to use. Most commonly, and for research purposes, adapted versions of the criteria for gambling disorder (recognized as a behavioral addiction in DSM-5) are used in questionnaires or scales to identify individuals who may meet the criteria for IA. The term *problematic internet use* (PIU) arose in 1996, and over the years it has been used interchangeably with IA. Most of the research done on IA comes from the Asian continent, mainly China and South Korea, where IA and IGD have been described as a significant threat to public health, to the extent that both countries support education, research, and treatment.

Overload vs. Addiction

Information overload refers to the difficulty understanding a topic or making decisions due to too much information. Over the past decade, information overload has become a growing concern in today's information-intensive society, given that knowledge and information are created every day faster than ever in history, and the body of knowledge and information continues to grow in an exponential manner. Currently, information overload, also known as "infobesity" or "information anxiety," is a problem associated with decreased performance and job satisfaction and increased work-related stress (Janssen and de Poot 2006).

When seen under the scope of IA, information overload refers to aimless Web surfing for extended periods, to the point that it becomes excessive and counterproductive to the individual. While absorbed in this activity, some individuals neglect other aspects of life, which leads to impairment in social, academic, and professional functioning. These impairments can often result in social isolation, affected relationships, being late to social events, being impaired or not getting enough sleep, poor school or job performance, not having enough time to complete duties, and loss of interest in other activities in addition to psychological issues described later in this chapter. Given the ease with which anybody can generate, publish, and disseminate content on the Web, much of the information presented to internet users is not entirely reliable. Although the ability of people around the world to share information is a positive, the downside is that the information may be biased, incorrect, repeated, or edited, posing the risk of misinformation.

Positive Aspects of Internet Surfing

There is no question as to how important the internet has become in recent times. It has emerged as an essential tool in many different aspects of everyday life, including business, education, academic research, entertainment, and communication (Davis et al. 2002). Constant advancements in technology have made it possible for the internet to continue reshaping and improving several aspects of daily life by being integrated into our daily activities. Every day, the internet becomes more available, and its services and uses continue to grow among every age group (Mihajlov and Vejmelka 2017).

For many, the internet has dramatically improved quality of life. Information is instantaneously available at the touch of a button. It offers unique business opportunities for online stores and restaurants and benefits shoppers, who do not even need to leave home for goods or services. People can manage finances and pay bills from their computers or cellphones, families can easily communicate with relatives far away with ever-improving real-time video calls, and virtual socialization continues to grow with multiple social networks, messaging applications, and even online games.

Although the positive aspects of internet use and expansion are very apparent, there is a growing concern regarding excessive internet usage behaviors. With continued growth of internet services and expansion of access to it, IA stands out as a potential threat for the future (Byun et al. 2009).

Diagnosing Internet Addiction or Problematic Internet Use

Kimberly Young (1996) was the first to write about IA, and since then a growing body of research and data has shown that excessive usage of the internet can be harmful in several different aspects of a person's life. Overreliance on the internet can be a detriment to a person's social relationships and mental health. Young described IA as being a broad term for a variety of behaviors and impulse-control problems. These are divided into five subtypes: cybersexual addiction, related to use of pornography and cybersex; cyber-relationship addiction, an overinvolvement in online relationships; net compulsions, such as online gambling, day-trading, or shopping; information overload or compulsive Web surfing; and computer addiction, related to online games (Young et al. 1999). Following Young's theory, Davis (2001) proposed a cognitive and behavioral model in which he made a distinction between *generalized* PIU, a multidimensional internet overuse not specific to any online activity, and *specific* PIU, which involves a specific online behavior.

In addition to clinical interviews, multiple clinical tools have been developed to measure or diagnose IA. One of the most widely used tests is Young's Internet Addiction Test (Young 1998), which is based on the criteria for substance use and pathological gambling. It is a 20-item scale that measures various symptoms associated with IA and their severity. Another widely used measure is the Assessment of Internet and Computer Game Addiction Scale (Wölfling et al. 2012), a 16-item scale that includes questions about frequency of internet use and negative consequences secondary to excessive usage. Fourteen of these items are used to calculate a clinical score and to distinguish from nonpathological use. The Compulsive Internet Use Scale (Meerkerk et al. 2009) is yet another questionnaire based on 14 questions, much like the Internet Addiction Test, about symptoms based on the criteria for substance use and pathological gambling. In addition to these measurement instruments, several other available measurements that are not as widespread include the Online Cognitions Scale (Davis et al. 2002), Internet Addiction Scale (Chen et al. 2003), Generalized Problematic Internet Use Scale (Caplan 2002), and Internet-Related Addictive Behavior Inventory (Brenner 1997).

Tao et al. (2010) went further in their attempt to develop diagnostic criteria for IA and to assess the validity of these criteria. To make a diagnosis, patients would need to have clinically significant functional or psychosocial impairment coinciding with the problematic behavior for at least 3 months, at least 6 hours of nonessential use of the internet per day, and preoccupation and withdrawal when not able to go online. They would also need to have at least one of the following: lack of control, tolerance (or the need for increasing time online to feel satisfaction), loss of interests excluding internet use, continued excessive use despite knowledge of negative effects, and using the internet to escape or relieve a dysphoric mood. These criteria are the basis for current criteria for IGD in DSM-5.

Given the heterogeneity of scales and questionnaires for assessment of IA in conjunction with the varying samples and limited studies, comparing the prevalence of IA is challenging, ranging from 0.7% to 26% across different populations (Kuss et al. 2014). Among Asian populations there is a higher reported prevalence of IA than in European and American populations. Younger age and male sex are considered risk factors, and most studies have focused on these populations (Kuss and Lopez-Fernandez 2016). Middle-aged and older populations have not been studied comprehensively. Females are also vulnerable to IA (Xin et al. 2017); however, it is unclear whether female populations have been understudied.

Comorbidity

In their article, Kuss and Lopez-Fernandez (2016) reviewed several studies of comorbidity with IA. Although it is unclear if the relationship between

IA and its comorbidities is one of causality or common psychopathology, it has been said that with a diagnosis of IA, comorbidity is the norm rather than the exception. In this review, they found a wide range of comorbidities; the most frequent was depressive disorders, with a prevalence ranging from 15% to 30%, and dysthymia, which ranged from 5% to 26%. Other addictive disorders, including gambling and substance use, had a prevalence of up to 26% in patients seeking help for IA, whereas ADHD was found in up to 14% of participants of one study. Anxiety disorders were also found to be comorbid with IA, with generalized anxiety disorder ranging from 7.5% to 15%, social anxiety ranging from 10% to 15%, and OCD with 7%. Personality disorders also showed higher prevalence, the most common being narcissistic personality disorder (22%) and borderline personality disorder (10%–14%). Another study reported that 30.9% of treatment-seeking excessive internet users met criteria for bipolar disorder, whereas hypomania was reported as 7% in a different cohort. As for psychological and behavior research, it appears that there is a complex relationship between IA and other psychological, social, and emotional issues; moreover, excessive internet users tend to have emotional problems and to be "sensation seeking" (Green et al. 2012).

Psychology of Internet Addiction

Like other behavioral addictions, using the internet in a compulsive manner provides the person with an escape mechanism to avoid real and perceived problems. Given that addictive personalities have increased rates of negative thinking, which leads to pessimistic attitudes and low self-esteem, this "idling" from real life provides some relief by allowing users to escape their own negative and pessimistic thoughts. This escapism leads them away from their self-perceived unpleasant reality and helps create a virtual self that is liberated from real-life stress (Li et al. 2011).

The motivations for excessive internet use have been explored based on specific online activities, given that problematic online activities relate to the individual. This has shown that the multiple online activities have different motivations. For example, excessive gaming relates more to escaping from reality and from loneliness through anonymous socialization (Kardefelt-Winther 2014), whereas excessive use of social media is used to improve self-esteem and confidence, social abilities, and social support (Smahel et al. 2012).

Research into this topic has brought up at least three different models, in which IA is seen as a form of OCD (Grant et al. 2010), an impulse-control disorder (Shapira et al. 2000), and a behavioral addiction (Fisoun et al. 2012), all of which can overlap to some extent. OCD presents as an intrusive anxiety that can only be relieved by performing certain actions. In an ever-growing technological era with wide availability of the internet, it is not uncommon to see behaviors such as repetitively checking email accounts, social network feeds, or instant messaging applications. Pharmacological treatment studies support the OCD model because they have shown decreased anxiety and time spent online with the use of selective serotonin reuptake inhibitors (SSRIs), which are commonly prescribed for OCD (Dell'Osso et al. 2008).

Impulse-control disorders present as an impairment in the inhibition of repetitive behaviors that may lead to negative consequences (Aboujaoude 2010). The impulsive trait resides in the individual's sense of tension before performing an action, in this case connecting to the internet, which is then relieved once the individual goes online (Shapira et al. 2000). Other authors consider this model too restrictive, given that factors besides impulsivity traits influence IA, some of which may be specific to internet activity or comorbid psychopathology (Billieux et al. 2013).

The addiction model presents IA as a behavioral addiction in parallel with substance use disorders (Han et al. 2009). This model is also supported by the presence of symptoms similar to those seen in substance use disorders (Chakraborty et al. 2010) such as excessive use, with loss of control, neglect of other responsibilities, withdrawal symptoms or feelings of anger when not able to go online, tolerance or the progressive need for more stimuli to achieve satisfaction, and impairment in social functioning. Neuroimaging studies also support this model because they have shown changes similar to those found in substance use disorders (Yuan et al. 2011): in particular, enhanced reward sensitivity, lower activation in conflict detection, impaired executive control, and lower cognitive control.

Treatment

Despite IA not being recognized as a diagnosis, excessive usage clearly can have negative effects on mental health and functioning. This has led to research focused on treatment and prevention. Due to some similarities with other disorders, treatment has been extrapolated from other conditions, such as OCD, impulse-control disorders, and substance use disorders and consists of psychotherapy, pharmacological therapy, or a combination of both, because these interventions have shown to be effective in decreasing time spent online and cravings and in alleviating symptoms of depression and anxiety (Winkler et al. 2013).

Because of the limited number of published studies on treatment for IA and lack of consistency in definition and diagnosis among the research, the evidence for treatment does not present any solid recommendations other than finding combined treatment to be more effective than psychotherapy or pharmacotherapy alone. This, added to the fact that most studies lack randomization and comparison groups, warrants further research (Przepiorka et al. 2014). Treatment goals should not be directed toward complete abstinence from the internet but instead aimed at achieving abstinence from problematic behaviors. If the patient can regulate internet use, this will result in improved quality of life (Cash et al. 2012).

Psychological Treatment

The most studied psychological treatment for IA is cognitive-behavioral therapy (CBT). This approach takes place over 1- or 2-hour weekly sessions and usually runs for between 8 and 28 weeks. Initial sessions focus mainly on the behavioral aspects of the patient's pathology, whereas later sessions gradually shift toward confronting the distortions and cognitive assumptions that promote the problematic behavior (Young 2013). During treatment, patients with IA identify affective and situational triggers associated with their addictive online behavior and learn how to modify them into more adaptive ones. In addition to addressing problematic behaviors, CBT encourages other stimulating activities not related to internet use that would compensate for the decrease of dopamine levels in the individual, ultimately increasing the effectiveness of therapy (Cash et al. 2012). Most patients show improved control and a decrease in time online by their eighth session of CBT and have sustained improvement at a 6-month follow-up (Young 2013).

Motivational interviewing has also been used for IA treatment. This approach is carried out in six phases and lasts between 15 and 19 months. It focuses on gaining control and understanding healthy use of the internet. Patients gain a greater understanding of the process to prevent relapse while including their family members in a more systemic approach. Having family involved in treatment helps patients stay motivated and feel supported (Shek et al. 2009).

Pharmacological Treatment

Although no guidelines for the pharmacotherapy of IA are available, several pharmacological agents have been studied, with promising results. Different classes of antidepressants and antipsychotics have proven to significantly decrease IA scores in several trials. The SSRIs citalopram (Atmaca 2007), escitalopram (Dell'Osso et al. 2008), fluoxetine, fluvoxamine, and sertraline

(Bipeta et al. 2015) have all shown benefit in decreasing time that patients spent online. The tricyclic antidepressant clomipramine has shown improvement in symptoms in patients who have co-occurring OCD and IA (Bipeta et al. 2015). Use of the stimulant methylphenidate by patients with co-occurring ADHD resulted in a significant decrease in time online and improvement in concentration (Han et al. 2009). Use of the norepinephrine-dopamine reuptake inhibitor bupropion showed significant decrease in cravings (Han et al. 2010) and, in a different study (Han and Renshaw 2012), in reduced scores on both the Internet Addiction Scale and Beck Depression Inventory in a group of video game players. Other studies have had positive results with naltrexone, a competitive agonist at the opioid receptors, and with a combination of SSRI and the antipsychotic quetiapine (Mihajlov and Vejmelka 2017).

Acupuncture

A Chinese study in 2017 showed a significant decrease in IA scores in patients treated with electroacupuncture alone and with electroacupuncture plus psychological interventions, both of which had better apparent outcomes than psychological intervention alone (Li et al. 2017). The hypothesized neurophysiological mechanism of acupuncture as a possible treatment is its modulatory effect on the hyperactive reward and habit systems (Wang et al. 2020). Strong data to support acupuncture as a treatment are still lacking, but it has shown promising results thus far.

Special Considerations

When treating patients with IA, clinicians should consider risk factors such as younger age and male sex. This does not mean that female patients cannot be affected, and IA should be suspected if symptoms are present. Understanding that no diagnostic consensus has been reached, we recommend that the following diagnostic criteria, modified from criteria for IGD in DSM-5, be considered when IA is suspected:

- Constantly thinking of past online activities or planning future online activities (preoccupation)
- Symptoms when patient is not able to go online, such as sadness, anxiety, or irritability (withdrawal)
- Need for increased time online to achieve satisfaction (tolerance)
- Inability to reduce time or quit excessive internet use
- Abandoning or losing interest in other activities due to excessive internet use

- Continuing problematic behavior despite problems
- Deceiving or lying to occult excessive internet use
- Use of internet as a means to relieve or escape negative moods
- Jeopardizing work or relationships due to excessive internet use

KEY POINTS

- Although internet addiction (IA) has not been established as a diagnosis, it continues to gain attention as research advances and is considered a public health threat in some countries.

- IA mostly affects younger males; however, women are not exempt from the disorder.

- Current treatments include psychotherapy and pharmacology, and some recent research has shown promising results from acupuncture. Better results have been reported with combinations of psychotherapeutic and pharmacological treatments.

- When treating IA, treatment goals should not be complete abstinence of internet use but abstinence of problematic behaviors and achieving balanced internet use with improved quality of life.

- IA is a problem that commonly presents with psychiatric comorbidity, with high prevalence of mood, anxiety, and personality disorders and ADHD.

Practice Questions

1. Which of the following statements is correct?

   A. Internet addiction (IA) and information overload are not a concerning problem.
   B. The heterogeneity of current data warrants further research and standardized criteria.
   C. Prevalence of IA is well known and shows low variability around the world.
   D. IA is usually an isolated problem.
   E. IA treatment goal is long-term complete internet abstinence.

Answer: B.

IA rose to concern in 1996, and information overload is one of its
main presentation forms (A); both are growing concerns around the
world. Because of the heterogeneity of criteria and sampling methods
used for research (B) around the world, prevalence estimates vary
widely within a country or a region (C) but are constantly reported
as higher in Asian countries. IA has a high prevalence of psychiatric
comorbidities (D). Goals for IA treatment should not aim to achieve
complete abstinence (E) but regulated and productive use.

2. Which one of the following treatment approaches for IA has the most
   evidence of being effective?

   A. Combined acupuncture and psychotherapy
   B. Combined psychotherapy and pharmacotherapy
   C. Acupuncture alone
   D. Combined pharmacotherapy and acupuncture
   E. Pharmacotherapy alone

   Answer: B.

   Research thus far has shown that both psychotherapy alone and pharmacotherapy alone (E) are effective in treating IA. However, studies
   have shown better results with combined psychotherapy and pharmacotherapy (B). Acupuncture has shown effectiveness alone (C) and
   in combination with psychotherapy (A) but still requires further research. Acupuncture has not been studied in combination with pharmacotherapy (D) to this point.

3. Which of the following statements is correct?

   A. Internet surfing is an efficient way to find information, often with
      very productive results.
   B. The more information available makes the decision-making pro-
      cess easier every time.
   C. *Information overload* refers to having excessive written informa-
      tion and not enough time to read all of it.
   D. IA is more than internet surfing because multiple different mal-
      adaptive activities are associated with internet use.
   E. Use of the internet for more than 4 hours a day is a risky behavior
      that could lead to IA.

Answer: D.

IA is a broad term for maladaptive online activities, subdivided into cybersexual addiction, cyber-relationships, net compulsions such as gambling, information overload, and computer addiction (D). Internet surfing may be a way to acquire information if done directedly; however, aimless Web surfing usually results in roaming for random information (A). Having more information available does not mean users will be better informed, because information (especially online) can be biased or incorrect, and excessive information can cause anxiety (B). Information overload refers to having excessive written or audiovisual information that impairs decision making (C). Online time is not a risk factor, per se; what is risky is the time spent in unproductive online activities and neglecting other activities (E).

Resources for Clinicians, Patients, and Families

Are You Addicted to the Internet? (https://psychcentral.com/quizzes/internet-addiction-quiz): Self-assessment tool to help identify unhealthy internet usage.

Center for Internet and Technology Addiction (https://virtual-addiction.com): Recovery center specializing in technological addictions that offers assessment, treatment, and intensive therapy for patients and education seminars and resources for professionals.

Center for On-Line Addiction (www.netaddiction.com): Website of Dr. Kimberly Young that offers education, resources, workshops for professionals, and treatment for people diagnosed with internet addiction.

NoSurf: Stop Spending Time On the Net (www.reddit.com/r/nosurf/): A community of people focused on becoming more productive and wasting less time mindlessly surfing the internet.

Zur Institute Online Course on Internet Addiction (www.zurinstitute.com/course/internet-addiction): Online course focused on how to assess and treat internet addiction.

References

Aboujaoude E: Problematic internet use: an overview. World Psychiatry 9(2):85–90, 2010 20671890

American Psychiatric Association: Diagnostic and Statistical Manual of Mental Disorders, 5th Edition. Arlington, VA, American Psychiatric Association, 2013

Atmaca M: A case of problematic internet use successfully treated with an SSRI-antipsychotic combination. Prog Neuropsychopharmacol Biol Psychiatry 31(4):961–962, 2007 17321659

Berners-Lee T: Information management: a proposal. Tim Berners-Lee, 1989. Available at: http://www.w3.org/history/1989/proposal.html. Accessed March 14, 2021.

Berners-Lee T, Cailliau R: World Wide Web: proposal for a hypertext project (online). November 12, 1990. Available at: https://www.w3.org/Proposal.html. Accessed March 14, 2021.

Billieux J, Van der Linden M, Achab S, et al: Why do you play World of Warcraft? An in-depth exploration of self-reported motivations to play online and in-game behaviours in the virtual world of Azeroth. Comput Human Behav 29(1):103–109, 2013

Bipeta R, Yerramilli SS, Karredla AR, Gopinath S: Diagnostic stability of internet addiction in obsessive-compulsive disorder: data from a naturalistic one-year treatment study. Innov Clin Neurosci 12(3–4):14–23, 2015 26000201

Brenner V: Psychology of computer use: XLVII. Parameters of internet use, abuse and addiction: the first 90 days of the Internet Usage Survey. Psychol Rep 80(3 pt 1):879–882, 1997 9198388

Byun S, Ruffini C, Mills JE, et al: Internet addiction: metasynthesis of 1996–2006 quantitative research. Cyberpsychol Behav 12(2):203–207, 2009 19072075

Caplan SE: Problematic internet use and psychosocial well-being: development of a theory-based cognitive-behavioral measurement instrument. Comput Human Behav 18(5):553–575, 2002

Cash H, Rae CD, Steel AH, Winkler A: Internet addiction: a brief summary of research and practice. Curr Psychiatry Rev 8(4):292–298, 2012

Chakraborty K, Basu D, Vijaya Kumar KG: Internet addiction: consensus, controversies, and the way ahead. East Asian Arch Psychiatry 20(3):123–132, 2010 22348866

Chen S-H, Weng L-J, Su Y-J, et al: Development of a Chinese internet addiction scale and its psychometric study. Chinese Journal of Psychology 45(3):279–294, 2003

Davis RA: A cognitive-behavioral model of pathological internet use. Comput Human Behav 17(2):187–195, 2001

Davis RA, Flett GL, Besser A: Validation of a new scale for measuring problematic internet use: implications for pre-employment screening. Cyberpsychol Behav 5(4):331–345, 2002 12216698

Dell'Osso B, Hadley S, Allen A, et al: Escitalopram in the treatment of impulsive-compulsive internet usage disorder: an open-label trial followed by a double-blind discontinuation phase. J Clin Psychiatry 69(3):452–456, 2008 18312057

Fisoun V, Floros G, Siomos K, et al: Internet addiction as an important predictor in early detection of adolescent drug use experience-implications for research and practice. J Addict Med 6(1):77–84, 2012 22227578

Foundation Inc.: Reddit Statistics For 2020: Eye-Opening Usage and Traffic Data. Foundation Inc, 2019. Available at: https://foundationinc.co/lab/reddit-statistics. Accessed December 15, 2019.

Grant JE, Potenza MN, Weinstein A, Gorelick DA: Introduction to behavioral addictions. Am J Drug Alcohol Abuse 36(5):233–241, 2010 20560821

Green CS, Sugarman MA, Medford K, et al: The effect of action video game experience on task-switching. Comput Human Behav 28(3):984–994, 2012 22393270

Han DH, Renshaw PF: Bupropion in the treatment of problematic online game play in patients with major depressive disorder. J Psychopharmacol 26(5):689–696, 2012 21447539

Han DH, Hwang JW, Renshaw PF: Bupropion sustained release treatment decreases craving for video games and cue-induced brain activity in patients with internet video game addiction. Exp Clin Psychopharmacol 18(4):297–304, 2010 20695685

Han DH, Lee YS, Na C, et al: The effect of methylphenidate on internet video game play in children with attention-deficit/hyperactivity disorder. Compr Psychiatry 50(3):251–256, 2009 19374970

Janssen R, de Poot H: Information overload: why some people seem to suffer more than others. Presented at the 4th Nordic Conference on Human-Computer Interaction, Oslo, Norway, October 14–18, 2006

Kardefelt-Winther D: A conceptual and methodological critique of internet addiction research: towards a model of compensatory internet use. Comput Human Behav 31(February):351–354, 2014

Kuss DJ, Lopez-Fernandez O: Internet addiction and problematic internet use: a systematic review of clinical research. World J Psychiatry 6(1):143–176, 2016 27014605

Kuss DJ, Griffiths MD, Karila L, Billieux J: Internet addiction: a systematic review of epidemiological research for the last decade. Curr Pharm Des 20(25):4026–4052, 2014 24001297

Li D, Liau A, Khoo A: Examining the influence of actual-ideal self-discrepancies, depression, and escapism, on pathological gaming among massively multiplayer online adolescent gamers. Cyberpsychol Behav Soc Netw 14(9):535–539, 2011 21332374

Li H, Jin R, Yuan K, et al: Effect of electro-acupuncture combined with psychological intervention on mental symptoms and P50 of auditory evoked potential in patients with internet addiction disorder. J Tradit Chin Med 37(1):43–48, 2017 29956903

Meerkerk G-J, Van Den Eijnden RJJM, Vermulst AA, Garretsen HFL: The Compulsive Internet Use Scale (CIUS): some psychometric properties. Cyberpsychol Behav 12(1):1–6, 2009 19072079

Mihajlov M, Vejmelka L: Internet addiction: a review of the first twenty years. Psychiatr Danub 29(3):260–272, 2017 28949307

Przepiorka AM, Blachnio A, Miziak B, Czuczwar SJ: Clinical approaches to treatment of internet addiction. Pharmacol Rep 66(2):187–191, 2014 24911068

Shapira NA, Goldsmith TD, Keck PE Jr, et al: Psychiatric features of individuals with problematic internet use. J Affect Disord 57(1–3):267–272, 2000 10708842

Shek DTL, Tang VMY, Lo CY: Evaluation of an Internet addiction treatment program for Chinese adolescents in Hong Kong. Adolescence 44(174):359–373, 2009 19764272

Smahel D, Brown BB, Blinka L: Associations between online friendship and internet addiction among adolescents and emerging adults. Dev Psychol 48(2):381–388, 2012 22369342

Statista: Global digital population 2020. Statista.com, 2020. Available at: https://www.statista.com/statistics/617136/digital-population-worldwide. Accessed May 25, 2020.

Tao R, Huang X, Wang J, et al: Proposed diagnostic criteria for internet addiction. Addiction 105(3):556–564, 2010 20403001

Wang Y, Qin Y, Li H, et al: The modulation of reward and habit systems by acupuncture in adolescents with internet addiction. Neural Plast 2020:7409417, 2020 32256558

Wikipedia: Wikipedia: Statistics. Wikipedia, 2021. Available at: https://en.wikipedia.org/wiki/Wikipedia:Statistics. Accessed March 14, 2021.

Winkler A, Dörsing B, Rief W, et al: Treatment of internet addiction: a meta-analysis. Clin Psychol Rev 33(2):317–329, 2013 23354007

Wölfling K, Beutel M, Müller K: Construction of a standardized clinical interview to assess internet addiction: first findings regarding the usefulness of AICA-C. Addict Res Theory 6(January):1–7, 2012

Xin M, Xing J, Pengfei W, et al: Online activities, prevalence of internet addiction and risk factors related to family and school among adolescents in China. Addict Behav Rep 7(June):14–18, 2017 29450251

Young KS: Psychology of computer use: XL. Addictive use of the internet: a case that breaks the stereotype. Psychol Rep 79(3 Pt 1):899–902, 1996 8969098

Young KS: Internet addiction: the emergence of a new clinical disorder. Cyberpsychol Behav 1(3):237–244, 1998

Young KS: Treatment outcomes using CBT-IA with Internet-addicted patients. J Behav Addict 2(4):209–215, 2013 25215202

Young K, Pistner M, O'Mara J, Buchanan J: Cyber disorders: the mental health concern for the new millennium. Cyberpsychol Behav 2(5):475–479, 1999 19178220

Yuan K, Qin W, Liu Y, Tian J: Internet addiction: neuroimaging findings. Commun Integr Biol 4(6):637–639, 2011 22448301

Social Media

The Self vs. the Selfie

Lukman-Afis (Lukmon) Babajide, M.D.

CHAPTER SIX

Distracted from distraction by distraction.

T.S. Eliot

Constructions of Addiction and the Social Media Character

Everything should be done in moderation. This adage cautions individuals on the potentially deleterious effects of obsessive and excessive behavior. In an age in which social media is often seen as a utility rather than a diversion, "moderate" use becomes difficult to define. Often, a common way for people to gauge their own usage is to compare it with that of people they know. This may give people insight as to where they fall on a spectrum, but does it really give them insight into whether their actions have reached the level of pathological addiction? How does one define addiction to social media? Life imitates art, or, in the case of social media, life imitates an online narrative. Michel Foucault (1990) posited the idea that societal constructs were created through discourse and discussion, and today these conversations play out largely online. He believed that people function within socially contextualized constraints while simultaneously reinforcing those social structures

105

through discourse. Our behaviors and interactions are informed by our social media presences, which become self-propagating.

Addiction is commonly seen as a dependency, either physical or mental,
on a substance or behavior to the point that its discontinuation would cause
adverse physical and mental effects. When viewed through the psychiatric
lens, paramount in the assessment of addiction is the investigation of some
type of dysfunction that is tied to the behavior. This is one of the main ways
to distinguish pathological behavior from normal use. Addiction does not
operate outside of a social context. Dysfunction should be assessed under a
contextualized lens. Hence, addiction tends to also reflect what is allowed or
prohibited by cultural standards. For example, caffeine is not generally seen
as a dangerous or highly addictive substance, whereas cocaine is. One of the
differences between the two is that caffeine is legal and publicly abundant.
Caffeine may also increase one's productivity, which is highly valued within
our society. For many, caffeine is a necessity to simply do their job and be productive in today's society. It becomes easy for many to overlook the person
who drinks 10 cups of coffee a day, including their morning "eye opener." On
the other hand, something like cocaine is viewed much less favorably even
though it has a similar (and admittedly stronger) effect than caffeine. Cocaine
is illicit, and possession or use can lead to incarceration or termination from
employment. Furthermore, cocaine is a taboo substance associated with im-
morality. The juxtaposition of cocaine and caffeine illustrates that societal
norms help differentiate addiction from nonpathological use.

Social media is difficult to define, and the number of social media platforms is overwhelming. The *Oxford English Dictionary* describes social media
as "Web sites and applications" (apps) that promote "social networking" and
enable users to "create and share content" (Lexico 2020). The *Merriam-
Webster Dictionary* defines social media as any "electronic communication"
in which users can "create online communities" to share content (Merriam-
Webster 2004). Overall, social media can be described as a platform used to
share and create content and participate in social networking. Some examples include Facebook, Twitter, Grindr, Bumble, LinkedIn, YouTube, Snapchat, Instagram, and Tumblr. Social media can serve many uses, including
helping people stay connected to geographically distant loved ones, date,
have casual encounters or sex, market oneself to potential employers, and
keep up with politics.

Social media has drastically changed the geopolitical realm. Politicians and
political outlets globally use platforms such as Twitter and Facebook to have
greater and easier access to constituents. Some of the uses of social media are
seen as nefarious, whereas others are seen as a necessity or convenient. For example, LinkedIn profiles help advertise one's skills to potential employers and
make job searching and networking easier for many. On the other hand, other

social media entities may promote more controversial activities, such as sexual encounters, gambling, and violent acts. Social media also encourages overindulgence, because updating your social media presence constantly is rewarded and sparing use is discouraged (Andreassen et al. 2017).

Although social media allows people to stay connected globally, it has other, more self-indulgent uses that may even undermine a sense of connectedness. Much of social media is, arguably, used to relay an aesthetic to others. This may be individuals showcasing their lifestyle or brands displaying the latest fashions. In this way, products and services become packaged as "ideal" or "perfect" for consumer eyes through social media. Platforms such as Instagram, Snapchat, and Facebook have become conduits for people to market their "best lives" to the public—that is, a place where people can show others their new outfits, nice physique, exotic travels, beautiful houses, and charming families. Social media popularizes what was formerly a more personal aesthetic.

In the past, mass media outlets controlled the images of what was deemed as ideal by portraying such conditions in sitcoms, movies, and commercials, but this has now largely been overtaken by social media outlets. Many assume that social media portrays a wider variety of lifestyles; however, "likes," "retweets," and "shares" reinforce social norms. This propagation of a certain media product is known as "going viral," which allows rapid spread and reproduction of the act or aesthetic. Although arguably less "repressive" than reality, social media has its own regulatory practices in which users can participate, such as reporting offensive or dangerous materials. However, it is ultimately up to the platform to act against any transgressors. Through action, or lack thereof, a culture is created that has unspoken rules for what is allowed or prohibited, and these may change given the platform you are using. In some video game–focused social media platforms, bigoted comments, threats, and cyberbullying occur with a great deal of impunity. However, on a platform such as LinkedIn or Airbnb, this is much less acceptable and highly regulated. Regardless, the cyber realm allows people to indulge in a concocted aesthetic that may be somewhat or wholly discordant with their offline character or personality. "Do it for the gram/vine/likes" are common phrases that encourage performing an action or impersonating an aesthetic for a particular platform. Indeed, many platforms have their own unique culture. Some may even become so engrossed in their social media persona and the discrepancy between reality that it affects their self-esteem (Andreassen et al. 2017).

With the plethora of differing platforms, people may indulge in the many different aspects of their personality (even to a grotesque degree) without having to feel censored in ways they may feel offline. Ironically, this may deepen internalized issues for some, given the constant shifting and tailoring of presented personas that one may have to display on several different platforms. Suffice it to say, it would prove difficult to determine pathological behavior solely based on behavior on a single social media platform, given the vast array of platforms available. From a psychiatric standpoint, a qualitative evaluation of a patient's psychological state in relation to use may prove helpful; therefore, one should closely inspect the patient's use of social media broadly. Additionally, an analysis of these interactions and the influence that social media outlets have on the psyche will prove important for determining potential pathological consequences.

Social Media and the Psyche

Some have said that social media is inherently self-destructive, but this view is perhaps too simplistic. Both the positive and negative aspects of social media should be considered to develop a more informed vantage point on social media's impact on a person's life and psyche. Excessive social media use is often correlated with certain pathologies such as anxiety, depression, impulsivity, and ADHD (van den Eijnden et al. 2016). Furthermore, people with social media use disorders tend to have a psychological dependence on social media similar to those with drug use or gambling disorders (Pontes et al. 2015). Efforts have been made to codify the criteria for social media addiction via the use of a clinical screening tool (Andreassen et al. 2017) that uses nine criteria to define social media disorder: preoccupation, tolerance, withdrawal, displacement, escape, problems, deception, conflict, and persistence (van den Eijnden et al. 2016). However, these nine criteria may, at times, reflect something other than dependence. The difference would hinge on the patient's reason for relying on the social media platform.

Individuals may engage in a subcultural aesthetic via social media platforms exclusively for gains in social and economic capital. For example, some YouTubers are paid to produce videos on things such as gaming, interior design, and political commentary. Often, these users start out by producing material to a specific audience as hobbyists. The pressure to produce content is low at this early point, and the authenticity and joy of the hobby may be preserved. However, once one reaches a certain critical mass of subscribers, YouTube may pay the user to continue producing such videos, with the stipulations that the user produce on a schedule and maintain a certain number of subscribers or views to maintain a steady fund stream. What was once a hobby becomes a commodified product that is being sold to the masses of social media. As a result, feelings of inauthenticity, corruption, and decreased joy or satisfaction with the practice may ensue (Andreassen et al. 2017).

Social media users whose online persona is mismatched with real life can become disillusioned with their actual selves. This may lead to a dysphoric mood or low self-esteem. The relationships built with this concocted persona may be constructed under false premises, which may lead to a condition of false intimacy influenced by concocted aesthetics, contrived biographies and online interactions, or a false sense of intimate connection via "likes" and "shares." The contrast of users' actual life compared with that of their social media personality's "best life" creates cognitive dissonance. Individuals may come to believe not only that their life is mundane and stagnant but also that it is depressingly abnormal. This may turn into a self-fulfilling prophecy as these individuals continue to be voyeurs while wallowing in their own perceived loneliness. The dramatization of social media can quickly become internalized.

Tools of Engagement

Social media has differing effects on people depending on how they engage with it. Social media outlets are designed to incite constant engagement and to promote behavior that will reinforce said engagement. This leads to obsessive behavior, which may or may not have a financial impact on the person. One technique used by social media platforms to promote this behavior is "infinite scrolling," which eliminates the need for pagination. As the user scrolls, new content constantly loads so that no breaks need to be taken. As viewers are constantly bombarded with newly loaded data, they may find it more difficult to divorce themselves from the material. If they do manage to divorce themselves from the material, this may incite anxiety in the form of what is called "fear of missing out" (FOMO)—missing potentially exciting or stimulating action on the outlet and being ignorant of hip new trends (Kuss and Griffiths 2017).

Tools assessing the degree of anxiety-inciting FOMO that comes from social media outlets have found that the sensation results in lower mood and life satisfaction while increasing engagement with the social media outlet (Przybylski et al. 2013). The apprehension that comes with social media disconnection may be somewhat of a withdrawal symptom that encourages consistent, compulsive, and problematic use of the outlets. Furthermore, this fear may grow into a fear of losing the tools to access the outlet (i.e., phones and computers), known as *nomophobia* (Kuss and Griffiths 2017).

Another example of an implement deployed by social media to incite constant engagement is "autoplay." This feature automatically plays videos when they pop up on someone's social media feed, capturing the person's attention and all but requiring the user to engage with the media. If users do not want to watch or listen to the video, they will have to manually stop it or turn the feature off entirely. If autoplay did not exist, users would not have to go out of their way to avoid engaging with content. They would simply just scroll past it. Autoplay allows for more time spent with media, which is one of the goals of programmers.

Social media platforms often reward users on a variable schedule. This paradigm reinforces engagement by offering rewards in a nonstereotypical and nonpredictable fashion. This type of variable scheduling reinforcement has been extensively studied in animals and humans and is used in gambling and lotteries. It has been demonstrated to strongly reinforce behavior even when it causes adverse effects on the psyche and has been tied to issues with gambling (Pritchard et al. 1976). Furthermore, as seen with gambling, social media use disorder may cause impaired decision making, as assessed by the Iowa Gambling Task (Meshi et al. 2019).

An example of variable schedule reinforcement in the social media realm is receiving rewards or privileges (e.g., higher status access to certain features) when one logs in to an app during a certain promotional period. From the users' perspective, the reward is given at random times and rather infrequently, which leads them to believe that if they are not constantly engaged with the app, they may miss out on these rewards. In this way, users are conditioned into constantly opening apps and engaging with them. If and when users do receive an award, they may feel a sense of pleasure that reinforces this act as good or even necessary. When other users "like" or "share" a person's status, picture, or other media, this also provides reinforcement. Users then constantly recheck the app to see if their "likes" or "shares" have grown substantially since they last checked. A substantial increase does not happen on a predictable timetable, so they may feel the need to consistently check. Before they know it, checking social media constantly is a part of their daily routine.

Social Media as a Refuge

Although social media has numerous adverse effects, it can also have a very positive effect given its capacity to allow greater interconnectivity. Social media may encourage people to interact with it in a way that promotes a certain degree of dependence, but it can also foster nurturing relationships and community. On several outlets, such as Tumblr, Myspace, and Facebook, people can create profiles that reflect their personalities and qualities and thus provide an outlet that may be difficult to find in their own communities. Shared music, artwork, and stories allow online communities to grow spontaneously. Those intrigued by others' profiles can stop, explore, and begin to interact, which could develop into a healthy relationship.

Privacy settings on social media platforms allow users to screen out people they may feel to be toxic and only allow those who are affirming and supportive to interact with them. There are also many online support groups for marginalized individuals who use social media in some form or fashion. Vulnerable populations, especially populations with certain illnesses, find benefit in using online support groups for emotional support (Chung 2020). There are many online support groups for people with cancer, multiple sclerosis, and even smoking. In fact, research has demonstrated that online support groups can help prevent relapses to illicit substances (Onezi 2018). Many support groups cater to a specific marginalized (e.g., racial, sexual, identity) community and provide a sense of community, belonging, camaraderie, and security for those who may otherwise feel isolated and invalidated. These online interactions may provide solace for people who feel stifled in their respective offline communities.

Social media provides important information to many different types of people and helps them navigate their offline environments more efficiently and safely. Social media allows users to find safe spaces both online and offline. For example, the popular social media website Meetup allows people with similar interests to connect with others in their area. Individuals can even find financial support through social media outlets such as GoFundMe, an online fundraising tool. Users have used GoFundMe to help them afford gender affirming surgery, escape domestic violence situations, and pay for expensive treatments for otherwise terminal diseases. These resources would otherwise be unattainable for many.

As with most technological advances, social media is neither entirely good nor entirely bad. It is a tool that can foster adaptive or maladaptive behavior depending on how it is used. Social media provides clear, practical, and even essential tools in an age in which technology has become ubiquitous. The problematic aspects of social media go hand-in-hand with the good. Practitioners can avoid overdiagnosis by acknowledging social media's utility as a tool for work as well as play.

Addiction, Habit, and Productive Use

Social media addiction is described as problematic and compulsive use of social media platforms that results in significant impairment in an individual's function over an extended period (van den Eijnden et al. 2016). Currently, it is not outlined in DSM-5 (American Psychiatric Association 2013), and the current definition reflects more of a skeletal definition of addictive behavior in general. This results in a vague and potentially subjective theoretical framework under which to operate. As per the working definition, use must be problematic and compulsive, but this alone is insufficient to meet the criteria for addiction. It must also cause significant impairment in one's life and be present over an extended period. This combination of symptoms encompassed by the definition cannot be an ephemeral occurrence.

Breaking down the definition in this way sets up a common scenario of how definitions of addiction may be misused. Many parents without a firm understanding of the importance of social media may believe that their child has a social media addiction and approach a mental health provider to confirm their preconceived notions. Parents may say that their child spends "too much time" on social media and that the child's "grades are being affected." Although concern may be warranted, it would be premature to label this child as having an addiction. Time spent on social media does not necessarily correlate with problematic or compulsive usage or even dysphoria (Pontes et al. 2015). If the child's grades alone are affected, this would only be one aspect of the child's life (albeit a rather important aspect).

In this scenario, the time course of the behavior becomes essential for determining whether an addiction can be diagnosed. The idea of time spent using, searching, or thinking about something tends to be equated with being addicted for many laypeople. Yet this is just one factor to consider in the overall picture of addiction. Social media can provide numerous benefits, so it is important to look at what is not being said in the scenario. Why might this scenario not describe someone who is addicted to social media? Nothing has been said about what the child is doing on social media. Considering the person's intended use of social media is imperative when diagnosing addiction.

If the patient mentioned in the scenario is actively interacting with multiple facets of the social media outlet, this is less likely to cause mental health issues and portend poorer outcomes. Active participation in social media has been suggested as superior to passive interactions with outlets because passive interactions portend an increase in depressive symptoms and severity (Escobar-Viera et al. 2020). Active participation can translate to use that is more productive for the individual or community and may increase one's sense of self-worth and importance on a larger scale. Passive interaction with social media makes one more susceptible to idle scrolling and mindless use, which may lead to more destructive and maladaptive behaviors online and offline.

Another unstated unknown in this scenario is the allocation of time—that is, when exactly the patient is using time to be on social media. The mere length of time on social media does not correlate with mood dysregulation; instead, the type of usage and how disruptive it is are what correlate with dysregulation (Pontes et al. 2015). Indeed, the child may be using social media during times when the child can be studying (which may explain falling grades), but is this disruptive to the point that it impairs the child's functioning? Is this addictive behavior or a reflection of poor time management skills? Using social media during one's free time is significantly different than using social media during periods when one should be working. Is social media use disrupting sleep, feeding, education, former interests, offline relationships, and offline extracurricular activities? If so, a much stronger case can be made for addiction as opposed to just habitual use.

Habitual use would be akin to social media usage that looks more like a hobby. Discrete time may be allocated to social media use by the individual. This time may seem excessive to others, but the resulting behavior is not necessarily drastically disruptive to the multiple facets of the person's life, and the person is not experiencing constant trepidation, anxiety, or unease with abstaining from use (Kuss and Griffiths 2017). Furthermore, with habitual use, withdrawal is less likely to occur when use is ceased for an extended time, possibly because the person is not feeling as intense a drive as would a person who is addicted. People who can still fulfill their duties but will turn to social media whenever they get a free chance are less likely to have an addiction to social media.

Are children as susceptible to social media addiction as adults? Children have many legitimate uses for social media, such as obtaining learning materials, advice, and informal tutoring from fellow classmates. This would suggest that even the manifested dysfunction that the parents were concerned about may not be wholly stemming from social media usage. What if the child is working on a personal media project that requires a lot of time to complete? What if this child is having an online relationship with another student in a different part of the state or country? Albeit discordant with the parents' expectations, these behaviors may not be indicative of a social media addiction.

If the child is engrossed with a certain facet of social media or has a particular motive for social media use, the issue may not be social media, per se, but what the platform provides. In other words, one may have to decipher whether social media is just a conduit for the person to engage in problematic behavior independent of social media usage. Just because someone has an engrossing relationship on social media does not mean that the person has a social media addiction. The multifaceted structure of social media may, in fact, clearly illustrate problematic behavior that the person already has while simultaneously fostering that behavior in the outlet. In fact, as stated earlier, active and engaging usage of social media (regardless of whether that behavior would be viewed as dysfunctional in offline settings) would argue against a social media addiction. Therefore, having an online relationship or endeavoring to create an online project would be considered active engagement with social media. This is protective from mood dysregulation stemming from social media and from exhibiting an addiction to social media.

Taking an exhaustive history and closely examining problematic behavior are crucial to ascertaining whether social media is the root of the problem. If a person becomes obsessed with a potential Tinder mate and begins harassing or stalking them, this suggests problematic behavior outside the confines of social media that is being enabled through the use of social media. However, if a person is enrapt with Tinder and with seeing how many people he has matched with or is swiping through many potential partners' pictures to the point of neglecting other duties, this may be more indicative of a social media use disorder.

Deciphering between social media addiction or habit and an underlying and unrelated pathology may prove to be difficult given that social media may provide so many different things to satiate a person's different appetites. One must proceed with caution when making a claim about a person's social media usage. It may be more productive to start out by distinguishing between the problematic aspects and the benefits of the person's usage. By doing this, one can weigh the pros and cons of the behavior to further delineate the etiology of the perceived dysfunction. Distinguishing habit from obsessive and compulsive use and analyzing the type of use (passive vs. active) are important. Furthermore, collecting themes in a person's social media usage and comparing it with the person's offline behaviors may provide a more thorough analysis of where the pathology may lie.

Treatment

Given that the notion of social media addiction is not well explicated at this time and a burgeoning amount of research still needs to be fully conducted and published on the topic, proposed treatments require further study. As with many other psychiatric disorders, cognitive-behavioral therapy (CBT) has been suggested as a promising way to ameliorate the manifesting symptoms of a social media addiction, specifically regarding the resulting cognitive distortions developed or enhanced through social media interactions (Pontes et al. 2015).

As far as pharmacotherapy, more research is needed on specific drugs that are beneficial for social media use disorders. Through extrapolation based on the treatment of similar disorders, antidepressants, antipsychotics, and opioid receptor antagonists have been posited as potentially beneficial therapies in conjunction with CBT (Pontes et al. 2015). More investigation is required before the success rates or special considerations can be known in treating social media addiction. Regarding CBT, special consideration of FOMO and nomophobia should be specifically addressed in sessions (Pontes et al. 2015).

Although this field of research is still in its infancy, preliminary observations have suggested that abstinence is not an adequate form of treatment for social media addiction (Pontes et al. 2015). This is contrary to many other forms of addiction, such as substance use disorders, primarily because no suitable substitute is available to help patients decrease use and social media is often required for work, study, or other activities. Controlled use has been found to be more beneficial than abstinence in curbing addictive behavior relating to social media (Pontes et al. 2015).

Allocation, intention, and mode of use are all important features in aiding with addictive behaviors. People should attempt to allocate time for social media much as they would for other projects, duties, or daily activities. If a patient and provider agree to set limits, the patient should abide by the time constraints put forth. Purely passive use, such as browsing social media to just view, like, and share material, should be time limited. Every time a person uses social media, it should be with a clear intention or goal in mind. Examples include connecting with a friend, posting material, connecting with an organization, watching an informational video, or checking in with a family member. Importantly, one must complete that goal and then move on and not get lost in the vast abundance of information presented.

Passive use (e.g., browsing, scrolling) should be highly self-regulated and given strict time constraints. Journaling one's use is a good way to turn passive into active. Recording interesting or informative things that one discovers during a passive scroll or browse may promote more productive engagement with social media. Because social media addiction is still ambiguous, the treatment options are not as robust as for other highly studied pathologies. CBT and behavioral modifications are currently promoted as gold standard treatment modalities. Complete abstinence is not recommended for people who may have social media addiction.

Special Considerations

Given the multifaceted aspect of social media, there are some special considerations when considering whether someone has a social media addiction. Social media outlets have proven beneficial for many marginalized groups and may be a prominent point for solace seekers from their invalidating offline environment. Hence, a seemingly large amount of time may be spent on particular social media outlets by these individuals for their own psychological benefit and as an escape from their invalidating environments. Manifested "dysfunction" under toxic conditions should be handled with care because patients may interpret providers' efforts as oppressive, which may lead to adverse sequelae, including psychological malaise experienced by people who live in invalidating environments. Social media has provided significant relief and aid for individuals with chronic pathologies (e.g., cancer, multiple sclerosis, and substance use disorders); like other marginalized populations, these groups may seek solace in the online social media groups to which they belong. Such support groups may operate as safe, affirming spaces and can be beneficial in many ways. Providers must proceed with the utmost caution when attempting to regulate behavior.

The demographics of populations susceptible to social media use disorder remain unknown. Sex and gender, age, and comorbid issues have all been investigated as important factors in deciphering risk, but no current consensus has been found. Theoretical models for the development of social media addiction have been posited, including the cognitive-behavioral, social skill, and sociocognitive models (Griffiths 2013). However, these models inform proposed treatments, and multiple treatments may be used at the same time. Hence, aspects of each of these models should be considered when treating patients. The cognitive-behavioral model proposes that maladaptive social media use arises from cognitive distortions and is amplified by environmental factors. The social skill model posits that those who lack self-presentational skills are more susceptible to social media overuse. The sociocognitive model suggests that maladaptive use stems from the expectation of positive results from social media use and that this expectation, coupled with internet self-efficacy and deficient self-regulation, leads to disorderly use. Multiple models can be used in the approach to a patient; providers need not confine themselves to only one.

Regardless of the model employed, controlled use—rather than abstinence—is the aim for ameliorating problematic use and symptoms. Understanding the utility of social media use may aid in presenting alternative behaviors to patients, with the goal of reducing dependence on social media. For marginalized populations in isolative and invalidating communities, providers should offer solutions that can propel patients toward their goal of reducing use while simultaneously maintaining a positive patient relationship. Modifying use of social media as opposed to admonishing or forbidding use is the goal.

KEY POINTS

- When deciphering the etiology of dysfunction, address whether social media use is the most likely culprit or is fostering independent maladaptive behaviors. Social media's convenience and abundance may serve as a conduit that nurtures other dysfunctional behaviors (hence, social media is not the real problem).

- Patients may use social media to indoctrinate themselves into social media culture, which may lead to dysfunction.

- Active use is superior to passive use because the latter has a stronger correlation with mood dysregulation. Active use equates to intentional engagement (e.g., purposeful communication/connecting, writing posts, creating media), whereas passive use equates more to mindless voyeurism and propagation (e.g., likes, shares, scrolling).

- Time spent on social media does not directly correlate with mood dysregulation and may be more a sign of habit than of addiction. Addiction has more discrete signs, including intense fear of missing out, nomophobia, and withdrawal symptoms. Habitual use looks more like a hobby, where discrete time is allotted for social media use and does not greatly interfere with life duties.

- Abstinence is not the answer and does not correlate with better outcomes. Controlled use is the preferred method when treating.

- Cognitive-behavioral therapy is being offered as a promising treatment modality.

- Social media provides a lot for marginalized populations. It has been proven to be beneficial for people with illnesses, marginalized identities, and addiction problems and may prove to be vital for those in invalidating environments.

Practice Questions

1. Gerald is a 16-year-old boy in the eleventh grade. His parents are worried about his social media use, reporting that he spends anywhere from 5 to 8 hours a day on social media. As a result, he has slipped from making all As to making a C in Algebra (but is still making As in all other

subjects). They have attempted to forbid Gerald from using social media sites but consistently catch him covertly using the sites against their wishes. They are now seeking psychiatric treatment for their son.

Gerald relays being in good spirits, even considering his punishment; he reports that he enjoys listening to music, playing soccer, and traveling. He estimates that he spends about 3–4 hours a day on social media, usually conversing with friends he has met while abroad. He also states that, at times, he will look at his friends' profiles to see where they have been traveling to. He also posts videos of his soccer skills on his page. Regarding his algebra class, the patient reports, "I hate that class so much. The teacher is useless and doesn't know how to do his job. Most people aren't doing well. I'm banking on a curve." Gerald denies any suicidal or homicidal ideations or perceptual disturbances. He is neither taking any medications nor has any medical conditions and is developmentally appropriate.

What is the next best step?

A. Tell Gerald and his family that he has an issue with social media addiction and that, as a team, you will have to implement a plan to extinguish his use of social media.
B. Start cognitive-behavioral therapy (CBT) with Gerald for his social media use.
C. Start dextroamphetamine.
D. Reassure the parents that this is probably not an addiction to social media and discuss ways of limiting his use to a healthier amount of time.
E. Recommend inpatient hospitalization.

Answer: D.

Gerald exhibits signs of possible excessive use of social media; however, he is an active participant on these platforms. Furthermore, his decline in one area could be due to many reasons outside of social media. He reports good mood and a continued interest in former hobbies. It is implied that he is using social media platforms to portray his hobbies to others and to interact with other like-minded people. Although he may benefit from more regulation of his social media use, to call his behavior *addictive* may be premature. Gerald does seem to be showing signs of difficulty in managing his time on and divorcing himself from social media, but, even if his use is largely problematic, total abstinence (A) would not be the treatment in this situation. There is no need for CBT (B) at this time because he does not appear to have cognitive distortions relating to his social media use. A stimulant (C) is not warranted because it is not clear if the patient has ADHD. Inpatient hospitalization (E) is not warranted at this time because safety is not a concern in this scenario.

2. Suzanne is a 17-year-old senior in high school who is brought in by her parents due to falling grades. She used to make all As but is now making a C in biology. She was the head cheerleader at her school but has quit because "I'm not pretty enough and don't deserve to be head cheerleader." She also recently broke up with her girlfriend because she noticed that the girlfriend has been "liking" pictures of other people besides her own. She bemoans the fact that she must continue going to school or doing chores at home because "my life cannot be consumed by this while other girls are living it up." She reports that she used to like cheering, volunteering at the animal shelter, and horseback riding, all of which she has since given up because "they are all pointless when your life is meaningless. I can never attain what other girls already have." When asked about her current hobbies, Suzanne states that she mainly spends her time scrolling through things on Facebook, Instagram, Snapchat, and TikTok "because it is something to do," even though these things do not particularly bring her joy. She even admits, "It makes me depressed seeing all of those other girls' lives and comparing it with my destitute life." The patient is not taking any medications and has no medical problems. She currently denies any suicidal or homicidal thoughts or perceptual disturbances and is developmentally appropriate.

    What is the next best step?

    A. Reassure the parents that this is probably not an addiction to social media and discuss ways of limiting her use to a healthier amount of time.
    B. Start an antipsychotic medication for paranoia.
    C. Discuss with the patient and her family that she may have a social media use disorder (with possible co-occurring depressive disorder) and may need interventions such as CBT, pharmacotherapy, and use regulation to improve her mood.
    D. Reassure the parents that the patient does not have a social media use disorder and that the underlying issue is a problem with her relationship, which is manifesting as anhedonia and melancholy, and that she will need to be started on a selective serotonin reuptake inhibitor (SSRI).
    E. Start dextroamphetamine.

Answer: C.

Several signs in this scenario make a social media use disorder or addiction more probable. First, Suzanne is having impairment in multiple aspects of her life, including school, hobbies, relationships, and her psyche. She presents with depressed mood and anhedonia and reports very passive use of social media. She attributes at least some of this mood dysregulation to her social media use, and it has also disrupted her relationship with her girlfriend. She is exhibiting signs of depression, with the chronic inciter being social media use. There is no indication for an antipsychotic (B) at this time because we do not have enough information to determine whether Suzanne is unreasonably paranoid about her girlfriend. Although she may eventually need an SSRI (D), to say that her current manifesting symptoms are all due to her relationship would be a grave oversight to the role her social media use is playing in her mood dysregulation and overall disenchantment with herself and her life. Furthermore, her issue with her girlfriend seems to be incited by social media activity, and we have no information about any other reasons to suggest an issue with her girlfriend beyond this. A stimulant is not warranted at this time because there is not enough information to suggest ADHD in this patient (E).

3. Johnny is a 30-year-old married man who is brought to your office by his wife due to her belief that he is addicted to social media. "He spends almost every waking moment on social media sites," she states in frustration. "Whenever, I go into his phone, he has Instagram, Snapchat, Facebook, and other sites I've never heard of open, and they're filled with cats! Just CATS, CATS, CATS, CATS!" she yells tearfully. She begs you to treat him for social media addiction. Johnny reports that he is a veterinary technician at his local veterinary hospital. He loves his work and reports it to be very fulfilling; he just got a raise due to his productivity. He is happy with his life and has three "babies," which he describes as tabby, calico, and short-haired cats. He reports spending about 6 hours a day on social media sites "looking at, producing, or commenting on cat pictures and cat memes." However, he exclaims, "I work, I spend time with my wife, I have a good friend group I see regularly, and I'm an upstanding citizen! Am I not allowed to have a passion?" He is not taking any medications and has no medical problems. He currently denies any suicidal or homicidal thoughts or perceptual disturbances and is developmentally appropriate.

What is the next best step?

A. Start dextroamphetamine.
B. Reassure the patient's wife that he does not have a social media use disorder and discuss the ways in which he can limit his use of social media to a healthier amount.
C. Discuss with Johnny and his wife that he may have a social media use disorder and that he may benefit from use regulation and CBT.
D. Further explore Johnny's use of social media and his offline hobbies because social media use may not be the prominent issue here.
E. Start an SSRI.

Answer: D.

Clearly, this man loves cats. Social media may be serving as a conduit to further his passion. He is not having problems at work or in many other aspects of his life. His social media use has proven concerning to his wife, to the point that she brought him to see a psychiatrist, but it does not seem to be disrupting his life in any other way. Given the whole picture as painted in the scenario, Johnny does not have a social media addiction. However, simply reassuring the wife and patient that social media use disorder is unlikely is insufficient in this case because social media is acting as a conduit to something that may prove to be important. Further exploration should be done regarding Johnny's possible infatuation with cats and whether this is an issue of concern. There is no indication to start a stimulant (A) or an SSRI (E) for this patient because he is not reporting signs of ADHD or mood dysregulation.

Resources for Clinicians, Patients, and Families

Addiction Resource (https://addictionresource.com/addiction/technology-addiction/social-media-addiction)
eMentalHealth.ca Social Media Screening tool (www.ementalhealth.ca/index.php?m=surveyandID=56)
Social Media Disorder Scale (www.psytoolkit.org/survey-library/social-media-disorder-scale.html)

References

American Psychiatric Association: Diagnostic and Statistical Manual of Mental Disorders, 5th Edition. Arlington, VA, American Psychiatric Association, 2013

Andreassen C, Billieux J, Griffiths MD, et al: The relationship between addictive use of social media and video games and symptoms of psychiatric disorders: a large-scale cross-sectional study. Psychol Addict Behav 30(2):252–262, 2016 26999354

Andreassen CS, Pallesen S, Griffiths MD: The relationship between addictive use of social media, narcissism, and self-esteem: findings from a large national survey. Addict Behav 64:287–293, 2017 27072491

Chung JE: Social networking in online support groups for health: how online social networking benefits patients. J Health Commun 19(6):639–659, 2020 23557148

Escobar-Viera CG, Shensa A, Bowman ND, et al: Passive and active social media use and depressive symptoms among United States adults. Cyberpsychol Behav Soc Netw 21(7):437–443, 2020 29995530

Foucault M: The History of Sexuality, Vol 1. New York, Vintage Books, 1990

Griffiths MD: Social networking addiction: emerging themes and issues. J Addict Res Ther 04(05): 2013

Kuss DJ, Griffiths MD: Social networking sites and addiction: ten lessons learned. Int J Environ Res Public Health 14(3):311, 2017 28304359

Lexico: Social media. Lexico.com, 2020. Available at: https://www.lexico.com/definition/social_media. Accessed May 12, 2020.

Merriam-Webster: Social media. Merriam-Webster.com, 2004. Available at: https://www.merriam-webster.com/dictionary/social%20media. Accessed August 31, 2020.

Meshi D, Elizarova A, Bender A, Verdejo-Garcia A: Excessive social media users demonstrate impaired decision making in the Iowa Gambling Task. J Behav Addict 8(1):169–173, 2019 30626194

Onezi HA: The impact of social media-based support groups on smoking relapse prevention in Saudi Arabia. Comput Methods Programs Biomed 159:135–143, 2018 29650308

Pontes HM, Kuss DJ, Griffiths MD: The clinical psychology of internet addiction: a review of its conceptualization, prevalence, neuronal processes, and implications for treatment. Neurosci Neuroecon 4:11–23, 2015

Pritchard RD, Leonard DW, Von Bergen CW, Kirk RJ: The effects of varying schedules of reinforcement on human task performance. Organ Behav Hum Perform 16(2):205–230, 1976

Przybylski AK, Murayama K, DeHaan CR, Gladwell V: Motivational, emotional, and behavioral correlates of fear of missing out. Comput Human Behav 29(4):1841–1848, 2013

van den Eijnden R, Lemmens J, Valkenburg P: The Social Media Disorder Scale. Comput Hum Behav 61:478–487, 2016

CHAPTER SEVEN

Online Shopping and Auctions

The Ease and Sleaze

Faisal Kagadkar, M.D.
Ana Claudia Zacarkim Pinheiro dos Santos, M.D.
Lancer Naghdechi, D.O.

When I shop the world gets better, the world is better.
And then it's not anymore. And I just have to do it again.

Rebecca Bloomwood, Confessions of a Shopaholic *(film)*,
Touchstone Pictures, 2009

Culture, Psychology, and Practice of Online Shopping

Cornflakes, eggs, and margarine: These seemingly mundane items entered history books as the first online store purchase ever—through Videotex, an online service accessible by telephone. It was 1984 in Gateshead, a small town in northeast England, when the shopper, a 72-year-old woman, completed the transaction by paying cash to the local Tesco delivery man. Back then, online shopping was not nearly as colorful and informative as it is now. With the advent of the internet and World Wide Web, online shopping grew in popularity: from making an online banking transaction to buying a pepperoni pizza at Pizza Hut's website, everything was suddenly possible.

In 1995, Amazon and eBay launched their websites, where they mostly sold physical goods such as books and electronics. These products, along with music, accessories, and apparel, are the most popular categories sought by online shoppers today (KPMG 2017). However, the relative sales growth in these segments is expected to be minimal, whereas other segments, such as household items and furniture, are expected to grow considerably. This trend points to an increased sense of trust in online shopping, especially from younger generations, and the belief that nothing is off limits in online shopping. Disclosing personal information online no longer causes fear and hesitancy, and the idea of purchasing a new couch from the comfort of home has become increasingly attractive.

It is therefore not surprising that e-commerce is a multibillion-dollar industry, with $601 billion of goods purchased by U.S. consumers in 2019 (Young 2020). This is an increase of 14.9% from the previous year, a pattern likely to repeat with room for exponential growth. According to 2019 shopping data, online shoppers spent $9.4 billion in a single day on "Cyber Monday," which solidified it as the largest online shopping day in the United States, with a 17% year-over-year growth (Adobe Communications Team 2019). Cyber Monday is the day of online sales that falls on the Monday after Black Friday—the day after Thanksgiving and the largest shopping day of the year. This term was coined in 2005 and is a symbol of the power and popularization of online shopping. Every year, millions of people in the United States eagerly await Cyber Monday, and some await its crowded and chaotic cousin, Black Friday, with even more eagerness.

Despite these staggering numbers, there are even greater players in the world stage. Singles' Day, an unofficial Chinese holiday, is the largest day of online and offline shopping in the world. The sales generated by Singles' Day is larger than the figures from Black Friday, Thanksgiving, and Cyber Monday combined, with an estimate of $38.4 billion spent in 2019 just through the online shopping portal Alibaba.com (Pham 2019). Founded in 1999 in China, Alibaba is the world's largest retailer and e-commerce company and offers services in various sectors, including an electronic payment service known as Alipay that is used by millions of Chinese and foreigners. Alibaba's opening event for Singles' Day—a gala starred with performances from world-famous pop stars and performers, such as Taylor Swift—further stirs this annual shopping frenzy.

Why does someone choose to buy a product online rather than offline? Although the factors involved may vary considerably among different geographical locations, age groups, and genders, research points to a few similarities across distinct groups: The ability to shop 24 hours a day and 7 days a week, to compare prices in a more convenient and fast manner, and to save time are among the main reasons a person chooses to purchase products online rather than in physical stores. In addition, avoiding the negative aspects of shopping offline, such as driving, parking, being in a crowd, or standing in lines, is an alluring factor considered by online shoppers when faced with the decision of whether to leave home. In fact, online shopping offers an environment of social anonymity, which could predict an association with mood and anxiety disorders, such as social anxiety disorder.

Nevertheless, consider the limitations presented by online shopping, which include the lack of a complete sensorial experience when buying a product. For instance, many people consider the ability to touch, feel, and smell an apple at a grocery store an essential component of a purchase. Others believe that buying a pair of jeans must involve trying it on for size and fit prior to closing a deal. Furthermore, window shopping—the activity of looking at goods at physical stores, often without the intention to buy anything—is considered a form of leisure and even a therapeutic activity to many consumers.

The COVID-19 pandemic amplified the best and worst facets of online shopping. Quarantined people around the world were able to purchase food, groceries, and medications from home, avoiding the risk of being exposed to asymptomatic or symptomatic carriers of coronavirus. With the lockdown of stores and restaurants imposed in many cities, shopping online became for many people not only a viable option but also the only possible means of obtaining essential goods. The culture of shopping nevertheless underwent important changes during this period; items such as luggage, cameras, swimwear, and bridal wear suffered considerable losses in sales, whereas disposable gloves, cough and cold medicines, and packaged foods emerged as the fastest growing categories (Jones 2020). Conversely, behavior such as the frenzied panic-buying of toilet paper and disposable gloves became common and led to these products becoming unavailable in both the online and offline markets or being overpriced by scalpers.

The Path to Purchase

Perhaps the next obvious question is: Why do consumers trust one website or company over another? What inspires trust and instills loyalty? The "path to purchase," a traditional shopping concept, might offer some insight into these issues (KPMG 2017). This theory suggests that a consumer experiences four stages in the process of purchasing a product. Those stages are more likely to be cyclical in the online sphere and encompass awareness, consideration, conversion, and evaluation.

In the *awareness* phase, consumers come to know of a product for the first time. This is made possible by online advertising, online reviews, social media, and simply by interacting with friends. In the *consideration* phase, which happens when consumers research the product, decisions regarding which product or brand to buy are influenced by price, promotion, and brand reputation. Subsequently, in the *conversion* phase, consumers decide where and when to buy the chosen product, and preferred website, best price, and best delivery options are cited as the most important factors in this decision. Finally, in the *evaluation* stage, consumers share their experiences online, influencing future buying decisions. Younger generations are more open and willing to share and even sell their evaluations online, which has the potential to be either informative or deceitful.

The word *auction* is derived from the Latin *auctum*, which is roughly translated as "increase." *Cambridge Dictionary* defines *auction* as "a usually public sale of goods or property, where people make higher and higher bids for each thing, until the thing is sold to the person who will pay most." This definition, albeit correct, is limited. The auction process, which involves a succession of increasing bids by potential buyers until the highest bid is accepted by the auctioneer, is known as the traditional—or English—method. Conversely, in the Dutch auction method, the seller offers goods at consecutively lower prices until an offer is accepted. Other methods, such as the first-price sealed-bid Vickrey auction and the reverse auction method, are also used by different sellers. Auction theory studies suggest that regardless of the method used, the outcome is often similar when a given method is applied in the right situation.

Live auctions were recorded as early as 500 B.C.E., in Babylon, where auctions of women for marriage were held annually. The most beautiful women would be auctioned first, and it was illegal to allow a daughter to be sold through another method. Auctions also served as a means for obtaining and selling slaves throughout history. Hundreds of years later, sometime in 17th-century England, a new modality of auction emerged. This modality was known as "auctions by candles," in which the duration of the auction was dictated by a candle flame, and the signal for the end of the auction was the expiration of such flame. Avid bidders would study the behavior of a dying flame, such as a slight brief flare up, to achieve successful winning bids.

Fast forward to the end of the 20th century, and humans were still placing bids, albeit no longer around a candle. Online auctions, which are auctions held over the internet, became a revolutionary way of bidding for goods and services, with a history similar to that of online shopping. The first online auction website, Onsale, was launched in 1995, closely followed by eBay. However, computer-based services delivered by cable television, such as the Videotex QUBE, were already a reality in the late 1970s and offered several services ranging from real television to shopping, gaming, and auctions. Nevertheless, it was only after the popularization of the internet that online auctions boomed, allowing an increase in the variety of products and services offered and creating the basis for the surge in a vast array of auction types and models.

Perhaps the most important change brought by the emergence of online auctions was the facility and anonymity brought by the internet. In fact, one of the key drivers for this market is the ease of bidding through online auctions, according to a Global Online Auction Market analysis published in 2018 (TechNavio 2018). Like the path to purchase observed in online shoppers, bidders can compare prices, research product quality, and read online reviews during the whole process of auction. On the other side of the deal, the internet made it more profitable for sellers to sell items that have low values, given the lower costs associated with using online auction websites.

It is estimated that the online auction market size will grow more than $1 billion between 2018 and 2022, with 52% of the growth coming from the American continent. The collectibles segment is expected to account for the highest online auction market growth during this period. Moreover, the use of new technology, such as artificial intelligence, is seen as an expected and welcome addition to the bidding process, leading to its optimization (TechNavio 2018).

The Modern Shopping Experience

The experience of shopping on eBay has been tweaked and modified over time. Some of the unique features of the eBay shopping experience may contribute to its addictive potential. Inherent in the process on eBay, or an auction of any kind, is the idea of a variable rewards schedule. Shoppers are unsure of whether their bid will win them the item. When auctions are won on an irregular basis, this behavior is reinforced more strongly. After winning an auction, the shopper is not immediately forced to pay and, in fact, may decline to pay at all, with little or no consequences. This may encourage shoppers to participate in auctions for items they cannot realistically afford. On the other end of the spectrum, the introduction of a "buy it now" button allows shoppers to immediately snatch up items if they are happy with the price or worried that the deal will not last. This may lead to serial perusing of eBay with little direction or intent, which, as discussed in Chapter 5, contributes to "information overload."

Amazon makes online shopping very appealing to compulsive buyers via various modern conveniences, including long return windows, free shipping, and a huge variety of items available at a wide range of prices. Amazon now even allows users to participate in auctions. Amazon offers almost every type of products, from groceries to automobiles, which encourages users to do most of their shopping in one place, and the site shows shoppers used items along with new items, providing more appealing prices for expensive items. Special credit cards give Amazon shoppers perks, such as reward points, that encourage them to continue shopping on Amazon.

Easy-to-use mobile applications for many online shopping platforms, including Amazon and eBay, make immediate shopping available 24 hours a day. These applications (apps) feature "one-click buying" options, meaning that the shopper does not need to put in or even confirm payment information or a shipping address to purchase an item. These apps also have daily deals that encourage customers to check daily or multiple times a day, increasing users' risk for impulsive purchases.

Study of the behavior of consumers—or bidders—has become increasingly more common with the popularization of the internet. People with traits such as impulsivity and competitiveness thrive in the online environment. Winning bidders have been shown to be considerably more aggressive and competitive than other bidders. Impulsive bidders, on the other hand, are more likely to be driven by the urge to buy instantly, which might subsequently turn into a compulsive behavior. The possibility of participating in auctions from the comfort of one's couch while clicking away any glimpse of self-control certainly has a reinforcing effect on such behaviors.

In theory, the different auction systems create an environment in which bidders can make rational decisions. However, strong emotional responses related to feelings of possessing the desired object lead to irrational behavior such as overbidding, a psychological bias known as *endowment effect*. Furthermore, objects viewed as unique or desired by a celebrity are often sold for unfathomable sums of money far beyond their real estimated value. Therefore, bidding, in its online and offline forms, is not an exact science, and passion frequently outweighs the rationality expected for such activity.

Addiction vs. Nonpathological Use

Online Shopping Addiction

Online shopping addiction (OShA), like the other technological addictions described in this book, is considered a behavioral addiction (Grant et al. 2010; Rose and Dhandayudham 2014). It can be defined as a recurring failure to resist an impulse, drive, or temptation to shop online that is harmful to self or others, ultimately leading to interference in multiple domains of life (Grant et al. 2010). However, authors debate the classification of such disorders as behavioral addictions, some proposing their classification as impulse-control disorders and others as obsessive-compulsive spectrum disorders, especially pathological buying (PB) (Black 2001; Christenson et al. 1994; Ridgway et al. 2008; Trotzke et al. 2015). Proponents of behavioral addictions cite the similarities in natural history, phenomenology, and adverse effects, and neurobiological evidence correlates with substance addictions (Grant et al. 2010; Trotzke et al. 2015).

PB, shopping addiction, compulsive buying, buying addiction, and oniomania are several terms describing a condition that can be considered as the "offline" variant of shopping addiction. Is OShA a mere extension of PB, with the internet's accessibility, convenience, and easy payment systems simply promoting PB (Trotzke et al. 2015)? Or are they similar yet dissimilar conditions (Griffiths 2000; Trotzke et al. 2015)? Conceptual models and empirical evidence point to them having both similarities and subtle differences (Zhao et al. 2017). Some of the differences could be attributed to the parallels drawn between OShA and specific internet addiction (SIA), such as found by Trotzke et al. (2015). SIA is defined as a behavioral addiction with a unidimensional use of the internet or of a specific app on the internet (Brand et al. 2014a; Griffiths and Szabo 2014; Laconi et al. 2015; Montag et al. 2015; Pontes et al. 2015; Trotzke et al. 2015; Zhao et al. 2017). Trotzke et al. (2015) conceptualized a model for OShA that was based on an SIA model by Brand et al. (2014b). They employed a cue-reactivity paradigm that used photos of shopping, shopping products, and other related cues to study 240 female participants. Shopping expectancies (e.g., anonymous purchasing, avoiding social interaction, product variety), shopping excitability (operationalized by measures of cue-reactivity/craving), and tendencies for PB and online PB were measured. The authors determined that OShA had distinct features from PB and shared characteristics with SIA.

Rose and Dhandayudham (2014) combined concepts central to the addictive behaviors and to aspects of the internet that may promote shopping behavior in drawing up their model of OShA. They described seven contributing factors:

1. *Low self-esteem*: Online shopping may relieve feelings associated with low self-esteem through the "reward" of the repetitive behavior or simply through the buying process, as noted in behavioral addictions such as PB.
2. *Low self-regulation*: Self-regulation or self-control is the capacity to alter one's own state or responses to stimuli through cognitions, emotions, or behaviors. Individuals with low self-regulation, coupled with facets of

the internet that promote low self-regulation, such as timed discount deals, pop-up ads, and one-click purchases, are susceptible to OShA.

3. *Negative emotional state*: At times of emotional distress, individuals are more likely to act impulsively, and the ease of access and instant gratification from online shopping may be used to alleviate that distress.

4. *Psychological enjoyment*: Individuals with "reward sensitivity" enjoy the rewards of shopping, and the experience itself is associated with positive feelings such as enjoyment and excitement. Both of these aspects could contribute to OShA.

5. *Female gender*: In Western culture, women are expected to partake in and lead household shopping and to view shopping as an activity to feel better and ameliorate negative emotional states. Despite excessive internet usage being associated with men, the female gender is hypothesized as being a stronger predictor of OShA than the male gender.

6. *Social anonymity*: The medium of the internet offers privacy, social anonymity, and an environment that promotes disinhibition and lacks usual normal shopping regulation cues.

7. *Cognitive overload*: Vivid interactive product listings, timed deals, notifications, and pop-ups advertising cause cognitive overload and deplete self-regulation resources.

Information on the clinical characteristics of OShA is limited. When considering a diagnosis of OShA, other psychiatric conditions that could be contributory should first be ruled out, such as episodes of mania that present with unrestrained shopping sprees. A few SIA scales have been modified to assess and diagnose OShA, including the Shorter PROMIS Questionnaire and the Gaming Addiction Scale, with the former proving reasonably reliable (Christo et al. 2003; Laconi et al. 2015; Lemmens et al. 2008; Montag et al. 2015). Another scale worthy of mention is the Online Shopping Addiction Scale, which views OShA as an SIA and uses the six-factor model of behavioral addiction (Brown 1993; Griffiths 1996; Griffiths 2002; Zhao et al. 2017). The authors found the scale to have high reliability and satisfactory concurrent validity, indicating a role of the scale in screening and diagnosis of this condition (Zhao et al. 2017).

Online Auctions Addiction

Online auctions addiction (OAA) can be similarly defined as the recurring failure to resist an impulse, drive, or temptation to indulge in online auctions that is harmful to self or others, ultimately leading to interference in multiple domains of life (Grant et al. 2010). OAA falls within the same conceptual models as OShA. To that end, it can be viewed as a unique behavioral addiction, a type of SIA, an impulse-control disorder, or an obsessive-compulsive spectrum disorder. A study carried out by Peters and Bodkin (2007) identified four themes of problematic online auction behaviors among eBay users: psychological distress, habitual use, negative consequences, and dependency/ withdrawal that posit OAA as a behavioral addiction.

The concept of "passion" and its influence on OAA was investigated in a study by Wang and Chen (2008). *Passion* is defined as a strong inclination toward an activity that a person likes, finds important, and invests time and energy in (Vallerand et al. 2003). It is conceptualized into two subtypes, *obsessive passion* and *harmonious passion*. The former refers to a controlled internalization of the activity, whereas the latter is an autonomous internalization. Wang and Chen found that subjects with obsessive passion were more likely to have OAA than those with harmonious passion. They also found that individuals with problematic internet use or PB were more likely to indulge in OAA behaviors. Like OShA, information on the clinical characteristics of OAA is limited. However, information can be gleaned from other behavioral addictions, especially in terms of management.

Positive Aspects of Online Shopping

According to the Internet World Stats (2021), 6 out of every 10 people in the world had internet access in September 2020. This translates to more than 4.5 billion active internet users and potential consumers of goods and services around the globe. Therefore, shops and auctions in their online form eliminate the geographical limitations imposed by brick-and-mortar stores, supply consumers with virtually limitless options of products and services, and give providers countless numbers of potential consumers.

The internet also offers people with limited mobility the ability to perform tasks, such as purchasing groceries, buying furniture, or bidding for a painting in a convenient and comfortable manner. Furthermore, because retailers are not required to pay for maintenance of a building or salespeople salaries, products can be sold for a cheaper price. The ability to compare prices from several stores and to save on gas and parking are other important factors that might ultimately reduce the amount of money spent on a product. In addition, online shopping and auctioning arguably have an advantage over in-person transactions when privacy and anonymity are required. The image of consumers buying sex toys while wearing their favorite pajamas at midnight summarizes the positive aspects of online shopping: it has the potential to be convenient, discreet, comfortable, economical, and timesaving.

Treatment

The overarching treatment models in addiction are abstinence-based and harm-reduction models (Carnes 2015; Carnes et al. 2011; Rosenberg and Feder 2014), and these can be used to guide treatment in OShA and OAA. An integrated, multidisciplinary, targeted, and multimodal approach that encompasses various treatment strategies could be useful in treating OShA, OAA, and any comorbid psychiatric condition. However, research investigating treatment modalities in OShA and OAA is lacking. PB, the offline variant of OShA, can be used as a guide in the management of OShA. Cognitive-behavioral therapy (CBT), especially group CBT, has been shown to be useful in PB (Mitchell et al. 2006; Mueller et al. 2008). Other therapies include bibliotherapy, which involves the use of books as therapy; cue-exposure therapy, which showed benefits in two case studies; and psychodrama, which involves role playing and spontaneous dramatization to investigate and gain insight into patients' addictions (Bernik et al. 1996; Gomes 2018).

On the pharmacological end, selective serotonin reuptake inhibitors such as citalopram and fluvoxamine have shown mixed results (Black 2007; Karim and Chaudhri 2012). Other medications, including anticonvulsants, dopamine agonists, N-acetylcysteine, and naltrexone, have been investigated in behavioral addictions, with mixed results (Karim and Chaudhri 2012; Mouaffak et al. 2017). Additionally, resources for patients could include financial conservators and Debtors Anonymous, a support group patterned after Alcoholics Anonymous (Black 2007).

KEY POINTS

- *Online shopping addiction* (OShA) can be defined as the recurrent failure to resist an impulse, drive, or temptation to shop online that is harmful to self or others, ultimately leading to interference in multiple domains of life.

- *Online auctions addiction* (OAA) can be defined as the recurrent failure to resist an impulse, drive, or temptation to indulge in online auctions that is harmful to self or others, ultimately leading to interference in multiple domains of life.

- Authors who conceptualize OShA and OAA as behavioral addictions cite their similarities in natural history, phenomenology, adverse effects, and neurobiological evidence correlates with substance addictions.

- Conceptual model risk factors for OShA include low self-esteem, low self-regulation, negative emotional state, psychological enjoyment, female gender, social anonymity, and cognitive overload.

- The Online Shopping Addiction Scale is a scale with high reliability and satisfactory concurrent validity that can be used to screen for and diagnose OShA.

- Individuals with problematic internet use were found in one study to be more likely to indulge in OAA behaviors.

- Research on the treatment modalities for OShA and OAA is limited. Strategies and modalities that have shown benefit in other behavioral addictions, such as cognitive-behavioral therapy for problematic internet use, could be useful.

Practice Questions

1. Which of the following risk factors is not conceptualized in the development of online shopping addiction (OShA)?

   A. Low self-esteem
   B. Cognitive overload
   C. Male gender
   D. Low self-regulation
   E. Social anonymity

   Answer: C.

   Rose and Dhandayudham (2014) conceptualized seven factors in developing a model of OShA, and they included female gender, not male gender, as more likely to develop OShA. They asserted that women in Western cultures often lead household shopping and use shopping as a feel-good activity to ameliorate negative feelings. The other factors of the model include low self-esteem, low self-regulation, negative emotional state, psychological enjoyment, social anonymity, and cognitive overload.

2. Which of the following conditions should be ruled out before making a diagnosis of OShA?

   A. Schizophrenia
   B. Dementia

C. Mania
D. OCD
E. Depression

Answer: C.

Although any psychiatric condition can coexist with OShA, it is imperative to rule out episodes of mania that can present with shopping sprees before diagnosing an individual with OShA. Currently, there is very little known on prevalence rates of comorbid psychiatric illnesses.

3. Authors classify OShA and online auctions addiction (OAA) as which type of disorder?

A. Specific internet addiction
B. Obsessive-compulsive spectrum disorder
C. Impulse-control disorder
D. Behavioral addiction
E. All of the above

Answer: E.

The classification of OShA and OAA is debated, with a lack of consensus. Different authors classify them as specific internet addictions, obsessive-compulsive spectrum disorders, impulse-control disorders, or behavioral addictions.

Resources for Clinicians, Patients, and Families

Debtors Anonymous (www.debtorsanonymous.org): A 12-step program modeled on Alcoholics Anonymous (AA) to assist patients with incurring debt.

Motivational Interviewing Network of Trainers (www.motivationalinterviewing.org): An international resource for training in motivational interviewing.

Psychology Today (www.psychologytoday.com): A good resource for patients, with down-to-earth articles on many subjects that offer different ways of looking at behavior and suggestions for making changes. Site is an easily searchable and free online resource.

References

Adobe Communications Team: Adobe data shows record Cyber Monday with $9.2 billion in online sales. Adobe Blog: Trends and Research, 2019. Available at: https://theblog.adobe.com/adobe-data-shows-record-cyber-monday-with-9-2-billion-in-online-sales. Accessed December 3, 2019.

Bernik MA, Akerman D, Amaral JA, Braun RC: Cue exposure in compulsive buying. J Clin Psychiatry 57(2):90, 1996 8591975

Black DW: Compulsive buying disorder: definition, assessment, epidemiology and clinical management. CNS Drugs 15(1):17–27, 2001 11465011

Black DW: A review of compulsive buying disorder. World Psychiatry 6(1):14–18, 2007 17342214

Brand M, Laier C, Young KS: Internet addiction: coping styles, expectancies, and treatment implications. Front Psychol 5:1256, 2014a 25426088

Brand M, Young KS, Laier C: Prefrontal control and internet addiction: a theoretical model and review of neuropsychological and neuroimaging findings. Front Hum Neurosci 8:375, 2014b 24904393

Brown RIF: Some contributions of the study of gambling to the study of other addictions, in Gambling Behavior and Problem Gambling. Edited by Eadington WR, Cornelius J. Reno, University of Nevada Press, 1993, pp 241–272

Carnes P: Facing the Shadow: Starting Sexual and Relationship Recovery, 3rd Edition. Carefree, AZ, Gentle Path Press, 2015

Carnes P, Carnes S, Bailey J: Facing Addiction: Starting Recovery From Alcohol and Drugs. Carefree, AZ, Gentle Path Press, 2011

Christenson GA, Faber RJ, de Zwaan M, et al: Compulsive buying: descriptive characteristics and psychiatric comorbidity. J Clin Psychiatry 55(1):5–11, 1994 8294395

Christo G, Jones SL, Haylett S, et al: The Shorter PROMIS Questionnaire: further validation of a tool for simultaneous assessment of multiple addictive behaviours. Addict Behav 28(2):225–248, 2003 12573676

Gomes C: The psychodrama in the addiction treatment of pathological gambling and buying behavior. Rev Bras Psicodrama 26(2):46–58, 2018

Grant JE, Potenza MN, Weinstein A, Gorelick DA: Introduction to behavioral addictions. Am J Drug Alcohol Abuse 36(5):233–241, 2010 20560821

Griffiths M: Nicotine, tobacco and addiction. Nature 384(6604):18, 1996 8900263

Griffiths M: Does internet and computer 'addiction' exist? Some case study evidence. Cyberpsychol Behav 3(2):211–218, 2000

Griffiths MD: Gambling and Gaming Addictions in Adolescence. Oxford, UK, British Psychological Society, 2002

Griffiths MD, Szabo A: Is excessive online usage a function of medium or activity? An empirical pilot study. J Behav Addict 3(1):74–77, 2014 25215216

Internet World Stats: World internet users statistics and 2021 world population Stats, 2021. Available at: https://www.internetworldstats.com/stats.htm. Accessed March 30, 2021.

Jones K: The pandemic economy: what are shoppers buying online during COVID-19? Visual Capitalist, 2020. Available at: https://www.visualcapitalist.com/shoppers-buying-online-ecommerce-covid-19. Accessed April 8, 2020.

Karim R, Chaudhri P: Behavioral addictions: an overview. J Psychoactive Drugs 44(1):5–17, 2012 22641961

KPMG: The Truth about Online Consumers: 2017 Global Online Consumer Report. Amstelveen, The Netherlands, KPMG International, 2017. Available at: https://assets.kpmg/content/dam/kpmg/xx/pdf/2017/01/the-truth-about-online-consumers.pdf. Accessed 31. 2020.

Laconi S, Tricard N, Chabrol H: Differences between specific and generalized problematic internet uses according to gender, age, time spent online and psychopathological symptoms. Comput Human Behav 48(July):236–244, 2015

Lemmens JS, Valkenburg PM, Peter J: Development and validation of a game addiction scale. Paper presented at the annual meeting of the International Communication Association, Montreal, Quebec, Canada, May 22, 2008

Mitchell JE, Burgard M, Faber R, et al: Cognitive behavioral therapy for compulsive buying disorder. Behav Res Ther 44(12):1859–1865, 2006 16460670

Montag C, Bey K, Sha P, et al: Is it meaningful to distinguish between generalized and specific Internet addiction? Evidence from a cross-cultural study from Germany, Sweden, Taiwan and China. Asia-Pac Psychiatry 7(1):20–26, 2015 24616402

Mouaffak F, Leite C, Hamzaoui S, et al: Naltrexone in the treatment of broadly defined behavioral addictions: a review and meta-analysis of randomized controlled trials. Eur Addict Res 23(4):204–210, 2017 28877518

Mueller A, Mueller U, Silbermann A, et al: A randomized, controlled trial of group cognitive-behavioral therapy for compulsive buying disorder: posttreatment and 6-month follow-up results. J Clin Psychiatry 69(7):1131–1138, 2008 18557665

Peters C, Bodkin CD: An exploratory investigation of problematic online auction behaviors: experiences of eBay users. J Retailing Consum Serv 14(1):1–16, 2007

Pham S: Singles' Day sales for Alibaba top $38 billion, breaking last year's record. CNN, November 12, 2019. https://www.cnn.com/2019/11/10/tech/singles-day-sales-alibaba/index.html. Accessed June 6, 2020.

Pontes HM, Szabo A, Griffiths MD: The impact of internet-based specific activities on the perceptions of internet addiction, quality of life, and excessive usage: a cross-sectional study. Addict Behav Rep 1(June):19–25, 2015 29531976

Ridgway NM, Kukar-Kinney M, Monroe KB: An expanded conceptualization and a new measure of compulsive buying. J Consum Res 35(4):622–639, 2008

Rose S, Dhandayudham A: Towards an understanding of internet-based problem shopping behaviour: the concept of online shopping addiction and its proposed predictors. J Behav Addict 3(2):83–89, 2014 25215218

Rosenberg KP, Feder LC: An introduction to behavioral addictions, in Behavioral Addictions. Edited by Rosenberg KP, Feder LC. San Diego, CA, Academic Press, 2014, pp 1–17

TechNavio: Online Auction Market 2018–2022. TechNavio.com, 2018. Available at: https://www.technavio.com/report/global-online-auction-market-analysis-share-2018. Accessed May 31, 2020.

Trotzke P, Starcke K, Müller A, Brand M: Pathological buying online as a specific form of internet addiction: a model-based experimental investigation. PLoS One 10(10):e0140296, 2015 26465593

Vallerand RJ, Blanchard C, Mageau GA, et al: Les passions de l'ame: on obsessive and harmonious passion. J Pers Soc Psychol 85(4):756–767, 2003 14561128

Wang C-C, Chen Y-T: The influence of passion and compulsive buying on online auction addiction, in 2008 IEEE Asia-Pacific Services Computing Conference. Yilan, Taiwan, 2008, pp 1187–1192

Young J: US ecommerce sales grow 14.9% in 2019. Digital Commerce 360, 2020. Available at: https://www.digitalcommerce360.com/article/us-ecommerce-sales. Accessed February 19, 2020.

Zhao H, Tian W, Xin T: The development and validation of the Online Shopping Addiction Scale. Front Psychol 8:735, 2017 28559864

CHAPTER EIGHT

Children and Adolescents

Codependence Between Youth and Tech

Muhammad Aadil, M.D.
Aitzaz Munir, M.D.
Lancer Naghdechi, D.O.
Yonatan Kaplan, M.D.

The most important thing we've learned
as far as children are concerned,
is never, never let them near the television set
Or better still, just don't install the idiotic thing at all.
It rots the senses in the head!
It keeps imagination dead!
It clogs and clutters up the mind!
It makes a child so dull and blind!

Charlie and the Chocolate Factory *(film)*
Burbank, CA, Warner Home Video, 2005.
Sung by the Oompa Loompas after shrinking
Mike Teavee, a child with a bad attitude seemingly
addicted to television and violent video games

Relationship Between Mind and Machine

Social psychology is interested in how people interact with each other and how advances in technology affect those interactions. Studying these interactions is important to understanding technology's impact on social well-being. For example, the most basic method of communication since antiquity has been face-to-face interaction, but technological advancements have produced many other options, including fax, emails, voice messages, and video calls. Although these technologies provide the advantage of global communications at unprecedented speed, their development reduced the need for face-to-face encounters, leading to increased social isolation. Aside from the utilitarian role of improving communications, modern technology also provides a realistic media for mass entertainment. The internet plays an important role in both entertainment and communications. As such, it is an important focus for research in social psychology.

For instance, Prashant Bordia (1997) at University of Queensland conducted a study comparing the psychological effects of computer-mediated communication with those of face-to-face communication. He found that computer-mediated communication has limited nonverbal cues that infer meaning and limited social context descriptors such as age, sex, or status. The consequence of technological messages being stripped of their social context is a possible distortion in the recipient's perception of the message—for example, a recipient finding the communication rude or offensive when no negativity was intended. Studies have also found that the human brain responds to certain technologies similarly to addictive drugs such as heroin, opioids, and cocaine (Widyanto and Griffiths 2006). Both drugs with abuse potential and certain technological applications (apps) are found to overstimulate the brain's "reward system," leading to excessive release of dopamine.

Excessive use of technology can also lead to stress in the human brain, with two major consequences. First, stress provokes the brain to release cortisol in the hippocampal "memory" neurons, causing severe damage. Second, this stress deactivates the prefrontal cortex, the brain's executive center whose job is to limit dopamine release and inhibit the reward pathway. With the prefrontal cortex's inhibitory safety lever impaired, use of stimulating technology allows for higher spikes of dopamine than the brain's natural baseline level. The brain subsequently develops a tolerance to the higher ambient dopamine, driving the person to repeat behaviors that will continue to drive dopamine release. This drive to continue engagement with "reward system"–activating technologies is the basis of the technological addiction.

Children and adolescents are particularly vulnerable to technological addiction because their prefrontal cortex is not fully myelinated and still in development. Children who are addicted to technological apps such as social media and video games exhibit "highs" and "lows" that are analogous to those seen in substance use disorder. These symptoms may cause marked distress that can snowball into mental health comorbidities such as anxiety, depression, insomnia, and poor concentration (Alavi et al. 2012). In 2013, DSM-5 (American Psychiatric Association 2013) published modified criteria to include behavioral addictions such as gambling disorder. This inclusion reflected our emerging understanding that addictions are more complex than simply substance use disorder and may be caused by behaviors such as gambling or use of technology.

In recent decades, advances in technology have increased accessibility to personal screens for children and adolescents. Each software update further modifies the user experience, with a goal of increasing apps' engagement so they can generate more revenue. In this chapter, we discuss the impact of new technologies on mental health and well-being in the younger population. We focus particularly on why these technologies are highly addictive, especially for the developing mind, and what can be done to manage the problem. Our focus includes internet addiction (IA) and its subcategories: video games, cybersex, and social media.

Addiction vs. Nonpathological Use

Internet Gaming

DSM-5 defines internet gaming disorder (IGD) as "persistent and recurrent use of the internet to engage in games, often with other players, leading to clinically significant impairment or distress." The disorder is included a potential diagnosis warranting further research. Although the name signifies online gaming, the problematic use can be both offline and online.

Video games have been a popular staple of the modern child and adolescent experience for decades. Children spend a significant proportion of the day playing games. This includes playing games on consoles, computers, cellphones, and other gaming devices. According to a national survey, 88% of children between 8 years and 18 years of age play games at least three or four times per week. Among these individuals, 8.5% show signs of pathological gaming patterns, and this disorder is more prevalent among boys than girls (Gentile 2009). A review study showed that the prevalence rates are highest in East-Asian countries, especially among males ages 12–20 years (Paulus et al. 2018).

Although video games are meant to be entertaining, people with underlying risk factors may spend increasing amounts of time playing games to escape from their personal lives. Pathological video game playing can interfere with relationships and meeting basic physical needs, leading to gaming addiction (Paulus et al. 2018). IGD was classified as a behavioral addiction in a systematic review investigating its pathophysiology (Burleigh et al. 2019). That review found analogies between IGD and substance use disorders in their similar impairment in function, dysregulation of reward pathways in the brain, and structural changes, particularly the addictive behavior's association with dopamine release.

Multiple brain imaging studies in school-age children and college students with pathological gaming disorder showed changes in functional connectivity, gray matter volume, white matter density, and activation of the ventromedial prefrontal cortex (Weinstein et al. 2017). MRI scans used to study the effect of *Fortnite* and other addictive games on children's brains found that the effects are similar to those of drug or alcohol addiction. The scans found that the amygdala-striatal system, the impulse control part of the brain, became not only more sensitive but also smaller in size to process the stimuli faster (Han et al. 2012).

Several studies have shown multiple comorbidities with IGD, including depression, anxiety, ADHD, impulsivity, alcohol use, bipolar disorder, and autism spectrum disorder. The most common comorbidity is depression (Paulus et al. 2018). IGD is also associated with poor physical, emotional, social, and overall mental health. Video game content is another area of concern; high rates of exposure to in-game themes may contribute to negative health outcomes. Most important are virtual portrayals of tobacco and drug use that normalize these habits to impressionable young gamers. Loot boxes are another major addictive tool that target children in these games. Loot boxes are in-game objects that can be purchased with real money. When opened, they dispense randomized in-game items, such as weapons, tools, or costumes (Paulus et al. 2018). The act of purchasing these boxes and receiving a reward has a similar psychological mechanism of developing addiction in children as that seen in gambling disorder. Countries such as China and Belgium have even classified them as gambling and established laws to restrict their use.

Internet gaming addiction has multiple implications for children. As a newly emerging addiction, its neurobiological mechanisms, diagnosis, and treatment are still under investigation. Multiple research studies are warranted to better understand the risk factors, pathophysiology, and implications of IGD and to include it in DSM-5 as a separate diagnosis.

Cybersex and Internet Pornography

Internet pornography and cybersex have been readily available and spreading since the invention of the personal computer and the internet. In addition to commercial or mainstream pornography, the internet provides a platform for multiple sex-related activities, including sex chats, online sex games, online dating services, and other sex-related content. Teenagers are especially vulnerable to using and overusing internet pornography and cybersex. Internet sex sites provide a digital forum for adolescents to explore their emerging sexuality and connect with peers who are doing the same. This exposure at an early age can be extremely detrimental to their mental health and have long-term ramifications. Studies have shown a strong correlation between early exposure to pornography and the severity of detrimental effects, which include

- Modeling of inappropriate behavior
- Emotional side effects such as feelings of guilt or shame
- Premature sexual stimulation
- Development of harmful attitudes toward sex
- Development of anxiety and emotional lability

Watching pornography can be very rewarding for a developing mind, and children can become addicted. Although there is no clear definition of pornography or cybersex addiction in DSM-5, compulsive sexual behavior disorder (CSBD) is included in ICD-11 (World Health Organization 2019). CSBD is defined as excessive preoccupation with sexual fantasies, urges, or behaviors that are difficult to control and lead to severe distress and negative impacts on health, job, relationship, or other life domains. Some researchers argue that such disorders may be classified as IA, sexual addiction, or a compulsive disorder.

It has been theorized that when a person watches pornography, a continued release of dopamine in the reward system occurs, leading to neuroplastic changes that reinforce the behavior. MRI studies showed a change in the volume of the striatum similar to that seen in several drug addictions (Love et al. 2015). Regardless of the mechanism, involvement in sexual behavior that is compulsive and linked to excessive online visual stimulation is problematic and can lead to multiple physical and mental health issues. Pornography addiction can affect sleep, cause psychosocial distress, and interfere with routine responsibility fulfillment (Grubbs et al. 2015). No national surveys have yet outlined the prevalence of compulsive sexual behavior or pornography addiction in children; however, a survey among senior high school students found that almost 78% had visited a pornography site, and about 21% defined their visits as "habitual." Another important aspect of the study was that 19% of the pornography consumers reported an abnormal sexual response, with 9.1% reporting it as "addictive" (Damiano 2016). See Table 8–1.

There are two subtypes of compulsive sexual behavior: *paraphilic* (sexual behaviors that are not considered as conventional) and *nonparaphilic* (including common sexual practices such as excessive masturbation, going to strip clubs, or watching excessive pornography). Orford first described nonparaphilic sexual behavior as addiction given the withdrawal symptoms including anxiety, depression, guilt, and difficulties reducing or stopping the behavior (see Garcia and Thibaut 2010). The addiction classification is further supported by continuation of the behavior despite consequences such as legal and marital issues, sexually transmitted diseases, and effects on daily life activities (Goodman 1992).

Why some people develop addictive sexual behavior is unknown, although it has been theorized that children usually develop maladaptive sexual behaviors secondary to stress, trauma, or mental illness. Children who experienced sexual trauma or abuse have been reported to display hypersexual behaviors. Socioeconomic factors, such as family dynamics and peer stress, may play a role in pathological sexual behavior. Cultural attitude and stigma toward hypersexuality may vary depending on the child's religious and sociodemographic background. Although there is increased research and consideration of cybersex or pornography addictions, very little data are yet available to evaluate, diagnose, and treat such disorders. Further studies are needed to illuminate the neurophysiological pathways underlying the sexual technological addictions.

Social Media

Social media can be defined as websites and online apps or programs that enable us to connect with each other and communicate using mobile phones or the internet. Some of the most common apps include Facebook, Twitter, WhatsApp, WeChat, Tumblr, Snapchat, and TikTok. In 2020, Facebook had 2.50 billion active users around the world, with 88% of users between the ages of 18 and 30 years (Facebook 2019). Although Facebook restricts use for children younger than 13 years, it is estimated that 7.5 million younger children have accounts nonetheless (Damiano 2016). A study by Kaiser Family Foundation found that children ages 11–18 years spend more than 11 hours per day on Facebook (Damiano 2016). A survey in 2018 found that Facebook is no longer the leading social media app among teenagers (Anderson 2018); most are more active on Snapchat (81.7%) and Instagram (80.7%) (Anderson 2018).

TABLE 8–1. Pornography addiction in teens: facts and stats

Percentage of males reporting exposure to pornography before age 18 years	93%
Percentage of females reporting exposure to pornography before age 18 years	62%
Average age (in years) of first exposure	Males: 14; females: 15
Females reporting exposure was involuntary	43%

In a survey investigating the perceived impact of social media use, only 31% reported a positive impact, whereas 45% reported neither positive nor negative impact and 31% reported mainly negative impact (Anderson 2018). Although excessive screen time increases with each app update, the survey results showed that only a limited percentage of respondents found the trend problematic. A study conducted by the Royal Society of Public Health found that Instagram and Snapchat were ranked worst among the social media apps impacting mental health and well-being (Shead 2017).

On closer inspection of the design and functions of these apps, their addictive potential becomes evident. Snapchat's "snap streaks" are a prime example of an addictive social media function. "Snap Streaks" are a statistic tracked by the application as a concrete measure of social media success akin to the "like" feature on Instagram or Facebook. Specifically, they measure the number of contiguous daily interactions between two Snapchat users. To maintain and proliferate the streak, a Snapchat must be both sent and received by the "streaking" pair of users. Failing to log even a single day of engagement with the streak results in forfeiture of the entire accumulated count. Resetting a virtual measure may sound insignificant or silly to adults, but for teenagers engaged in the app, the streak represents a vested measure of social capital. Some teenagers may value it as a proxy for emotional validation or connectedness with their Snapchat partners. Losing a streak can be emotionally devastating, be interpreted as rejection or abandonment, and even catalyze dissolution of friendships. When teenagers' ego is dependent on external validation via the social media followers, streaks, and snaps they receive, their interpersonal relationships suffer at the expense of maintaining their electronic profile.

Social media addiction has severe implications for the mental health and well-being of children and adolescents. Excessive use has been linked to higher rates of anxiety and depression, low self-esteem, loneliness, poor community involvement, and poor academic performance. There is a strong positive correlation between time spent on social media apps and symptoms of depression (Pantic 2014). More research is clearly needed, but social media addiction is a widely prevalent problem and, in many circumstances, requires professional treatment. College and school campuses must screen students for depression related to social media use to prevent maladaptive behavior and offer early treatment.

Treatment

When to Screen for Technological Addiction

Technological addiction can lead to poor rapport of children with parents and other siblings, leading to distrust and dishonesty. Severe problems can lead to social withdrawal and trouble maintaining relationships as the person finds more comfort in the online environment than the real one, which leads to a vicious circle. Following are signs and symptoms of technological addictions to screen for in children (Sigman 2014):

- Sense of loss or feeling of severe anxiety when without phone or other devices
- Reliance on online feedback, such as comments, likes, or snaps for self-esteem
- Placing too much importance on social media apps and receiving vitriol online
- Insomnia secondary to excessive screen time
- Emotionally distraught or labile when separated from devices
- Obsessively checking apps for notifications
- Hypersexual behavior, vocabulary, and attitude
- Overprotective of technology, such as cellphones
- Isolative behavior and staying up late at night with cellphone or tablet

Psychological Approaches

One approach is relative therapy, which is a form of cognitive-behavioral therapy (CBT). In relative therapy, the focus is on present circumstances and relationships while avoiding problematic past experiences. Patients are presented with the idea that addiction is a choice and are trained in time management and how to solve problematic behavior. Relative therapy not only focuses on the addictive behavior around internet and technology but also on food and sex addiction. Studies have reported that it not only decreases addictive behavior but also is highly effective for improving self-esteem among college students (Kim 2008).

Acceptance and commitment therapy (ACT) was developed by Steven Hayes in 2011. Similar to dialectical behavior therapy, ACT is considered a hybrid form of CBT that emphasizes Eastern meditative skills and mindfulness while also focusing on cognitive diffusion. It encourages patients to accept their thoughts and feelings as they are, without assigning any importance to them. For example, a patient practicing ACT for video game addiction learns to recognize the thought "I am having a craving to play *Red Dead Redemption* again. I know it will be fun" and allow that thought to pass without acting on it. This exercise also provides a way for patients with gaming addiction and IA to fully experience their present without attachment to specific thoughts or events (Kim 2008).

Family therapy is another option with proven efficacy for IA. A multilevel intervention-based family therapy for early and late adolescents that included motivational interviewing, career plan development, behavioral contracting, and family therapy showed significant reduction in addiction severity after 15–19 months (Shek et al. 2009). Another study compared six-session multifamily-based therapy with a waitlist control condition (Park et al. 2008). The authors focused on building a relationship between the child and the parents around their IA through general communication. They attempted to find the association between unmet needs during childhood and excessive internet use and worked to establish healthy family dynamics. After 6 weeks of therapy, the family-based intervention was found to significantly decrease the addiction severity score and had the added benefit of improving the family relationship.

Multiple CBTs provide help for patients with internet, gaming, or pornography addiction. CBT is effective in helping patients realize their addictive feelings and actions, adopt new coping skills, and develop methods to prevent relapse. CBT takes 3–12 months of continuous treatment to appreciate an effect. The therapist focuses on the patient's pattern of use (e.g., excessive gaming or social media use), develops a new schedule to disrupt that pattern, and helps the patient set new goals to improve well-being.

CBT for IA (CBT-IA) provides a comprehensive approach through three different phases: 1) behavioral modification, 2) cognitive reconstruction, and 3) harm reduction therapy. CBT is a first-line treatment for IA and gaming addiction in children, with evidence from multiple studies supporting its efficacy (Zajac et al. 2017). One study conducted by Young (2007) that investigated treatment options for IA in 114 subjects found that CBT helped participants become motivated to seek help for their addiction, enhanced their motivation to stop excessive internet use, limited their computer and online pornography use, and improved their focus to obtain sobriety from problematic online use (Ong and Tan 2014).

Cao and Su (2007) also found that CBT significantly lowered addiction scores in middle-school students with IA. The students also showed significant improvement in psychological function (Cash et al. 2012). Multimodal treatment approaches are also being examined, with involvement of psychotherapy, pharmacotherapy, and family counseling simultaneously. This idea is supported by a long-term study by Du et al. (2010), who studied the effects of such treatment modalities on adolescents and found significant improvement in emotional regulation, behavior, and self-management style.

Pharmacological Treatment

The role of antidepressants, particularly selective serotonin reuptake inhibitors (SSRIs), has been studied because of the role aminergic systems play in repressing inhibitory responses and controlling compulsive repetitive behavior. Data suggest a high lifetime prevalence of major depressive disorder in patients with IA and gaming addiction. Multiple studies have also shown a close relationship between impulsivity, serotonergic dysfunction, and obsessive-compulsive symptoms, all of which may be treated with serotonergic drugs (Yen et al. 2007).

Another study recruited adolescents and adults and compared the efficacy of bupropion and escitalopram and found both were beneficial in improving attention and impulsivity. Bupropion was found to have superior effect in IGD (Song et al. 2016). Bupropion 300 mg was studied in adolescents and adults with IGD ages 16–29 years and significantly helped cue-induced brain activity and cravings for playing (Nam et al. 2017). Another study of bupropion 150–300 mg along with psychoeducation in patients ages 13–42 years showed that Beck Depression Inventory and Clinical Global Impression–Severity scores were significantly better in the bupropion group compared with the placebo group (Han et al. 2012). Another study that combined 8 weeks of CBT for problematic online gaming with 8 weeks of bupropion 150–300 mg helped with excessive internet gaming and the depressive state (Nakayama et al. 2017). Brain activity response measured with functional MRI showed that after 6 weeks of treatment with bupropion, total brain activity was lowered in correlation with decreased craving and time spent playing games. Antidepressant anticraving properties are not yet fully understood and are a topic for further investigation.

KEY POINTS

- Excessive or unskilled internet use among children and adolescents has the potential to develop into a behavioral addiction. This can have a negative impact on their psychological, physical, social, and developmental well-being.

- Addiction related to technology (internet, pornography, or social media) leads to excessive dopamine release in the reward system, and the neuroplastic changes are similar to those seen in substance use disorders.

- Internet-related addiction in children leads to high rates of comorbid depression, anxiety, ADHD, and substance use disorders.

- Major risk factors include various personality traits such as impulsivity, sensation-seeking behavior, low parental monitoring, family conflicts, and male gender.

- Clinical management includes treatment of comorbid conditions, cognitive-behavioral therapy, family therapy, and group therapy, and some preliminary studies have reported success with selective serotonin reuptake inhibitors and bupropion.

Practice Questions

1. A 13-year-old boy named John has been spending more than 12 hours a day on his iPad playing *Plants vs. Zombies* and *Alto's Adventure*. He also uses Facebook and Snapchat and responds to about 120 notifications in a day. His grades have been declining for the past 6 months, and his mother reports that his mood has become more irritable. After they had an argument, the mother took away John's iPad and cellphone and restricted their use to 1 hour daily. For the next 3 days, he continued to isolate himself in his room and had decreased appetite, poor focus, restlessness, and crying spells. He continued to become extremely irritable and agitated to a point that his mother decided to take him to a child psychiatrist.

What would be first-line treatment?

A. Escitalopram
B. Valproate
C. Lorazepam
D. Cognitive-behavioral therapy (CBT)
E. Dialectical behavior therapy

Answer: D.

John has internet addiction (IA) and is likely experiencing symptoms of withdrawal (irritable mood, restlessness, decreased appetite, poor focus) from having his devices taken away. Best initial treatment will be modified CBT for IA so that he can develop insight into the problem and manage his screen time. Dialectical behavior therapy (E) is the main empirically supported treatment for borderline personality disorder. Escitalopram (A) can be considered in cases of severe IA as an adjuvant along with CBT because it helps with anxiety, depression, and impulse control; however, in mild IA this should not be the first-line treatment because of its side effects. Valproate (B) is used in the management of severe mood disorder. Lorazepam (C) will only help with acute agitation or aggression.

2. A 15-year-old boy reports to a psychiatrist that he has been watching pornographic heterosexual content online 12–15 times per day. He says that his first sexual encounter was with a slightly older consenting female when he was 14. He reports that he has not been able to focus on his studies, has declining grades, and "can't think of anything other than sex." He frequently masturbates multiple times during the day. He also experiences anxiety and is becoming more socially withdrawn.

   What changes have been seen in preliminary studies on the MRI of patients with pornography addiction and are likely to be seen in this patient?

   A. Increased ventricular size
   B. Volume changes in striatum
   C. Cerebral atrophy
   D. Lesion in striatothalamocortical circuit
   E. Frontal lobe atrophy

   Answer: B.

In the scenario, the patient has an internet pornography addiction that is affecting his well-being and social life. An MRI will likely show volume changes in the striatum similar to that in several addictions. Increased ventricular size (A) is seen in patients with hydrocephalus. Cerebral (C) and frontal lobe (E) atrophy are features of Alzheimer's disease, and damage in the striatothalamocortical circuit (D) occurs in Parkinson's disease.

3. Jack is a 13-year-old boy who spends most of his time online using Facebook and playing video games. He struggles to go to school and misses his homework frequently. He tends to procrastinate and spends time on the internet instead of completing his homework. He mostly begins sleep at 2 A.M. after spending 4–5 hours playing video games. This has led to increasing conflicts at home. He has been diagnosed with generalized anxiety disorder by his therapist.

   What are the risk factors for IA in children and adolescents?

   A. Male gender
   B. Low family monitoring
   C. Smoking and drug use
   D. Impulsive behavior
   E. All of the above

   Answer: E.

   Studies have consistently shown that males are at higher risk of IA. Family dysfunction and conflicts and low monitoring of children often lead to either problematic internet use or IA. People with certain personality traits (e.g., impulsivity, sensation seeking) are at higher risk compared with general population.

Resources for Clinicians

Internet Sex Screening Test (www.ncbi.nlm.nih.gov/pubmed/21044551)
Social Media Disorder Scale (www.sciencedirect.com/science/article/pii/S0747563216302059)
Videogame Addiction Scale for Children (www.ncbi.nlm.nih.gov/pmc/articles/PMC5529472)
Young's Internet Addiction Test (www.ncbi.nlm.nih.gov/pmc/articles/PMC6198603)

References

Alavi SS, Ferdosi M, Jannatifard F, et al: Behavioral addiction versus substance addiction: correspondence of psychiatric and psychological views. Int J Prev Med 3(4):290–294, 2012 22624087

American Psychiatric Association: Diagnostic and Statistical Manual of Mental Disorders, 5th Edition. Arlington, VA, American Psychiatric Association, 2013

Anderson M: Teens, social media and technology 2018. Pew Research Center: Internet, Science and Tech (blog), 2018. Available at: https://www.pewresearch.org/internet/2018/05/31/teens-social-media-technology-2018. Accessed May 31, 2018.

Bordia P: Face-to-face versus computer-mediated communication: a synthesis of the empirical literature. J Bus Commun 34:99–118, 1997

Burleigh TL, Griffiths MD, Sumich A, et al: A systematic review of the co-occurrence of gaming disorder and other potentially addictive behaviors. Curr Addict Rep 6(4):383–401, 2019

Cao F, Su L: Internet addiction among Chinese adolescents: prevalence and psychological features. Child Care Health Dev 33(3):275–281, 2007 17439441

Cash H, Rae CD, Steel AH, Winkler A: Internet addiction: a brief summary of research and practice. Curr Psychiatry Rev 8(4):292–298, 2012 23125561

Damiano P: Adolescents and web porn: a new era of sexuality. Int J Adolesc Med Health 28(2):169–173, 2016 26251980

Du Y-S, Jiang W, Vance A: Longer term effect of randomized, controlled group cognitive behavioural therapy for internet addiction in adolescent students in Shanghai. Aust NZ J Psychiatry 44(2):129–134, 2010

Facebook: Facebook reports fourth quarter and full year 2019 results. PRNewswire, 2019. Available at: https://www.prnewswire.com/news-releases/facebook-reports-fourth-quarter-and-full-year-2019-results-300995616.html. Accessed March 2021.

Garcia FD, Thibaut F: Sexual addictions. Am J Drug Alcohol Abuse 36(5):254–260, 2010 20666699

Gentile D: Pathological video-game use among youth ages 8 to 18: a national study. Psychol Sci 20(5):594–602, 2009 19476590

Goodman A: Sexual addiction: designation and treatment. J Sex Marital Ther 18(4):303–314, 1992 1291701

Grubbs JB, Volk F, Exline JJ, Pargament KI: Internet pornography use: perceived addiction, psychological distress, and the validation of a brief measure. J Sex Marital Ther 41(1):83–106, 2015 24341869

Han DH, Lyoo IK, Renshaw PF: Differential regional gray matter volumes in patients with on-line game addiction and professional gamers. J Psychiatr Res 46(4):507–515, 2012 22277302

Kim J-U: The effect of a R/T group counseling program on the internet addiction level and self-esteem of internet addiction university students. International Journal of Reality Therapy 27(2):4–12, 2008

Love T, Laier C, Brand M, et al: Neuroscience of internet pornography addiction: a review and update. Behav Sci (Basel) 5(3):388–433, 2015 26393658

Nakayama H, Mihara S, Higuchi S: Treatment and risk factors of internet use disorders. Psychiatry Clin Neurosci 71(7):492–505, 2017 27987253

Nam B, Bae S, Kim SM, et al: Comparing the effects of bupropion and escitalopram on excessive internet game play in patients with major depressive disorder. Clin Psychopharmacol Neurosci 15(4):361–368, 2017 29073748

Ong SH, Tan YR: Internet addiction in young people. Ann Acad Med Singapore 43(7):378–382, 2014 25142474

Pantic I: Online social networking and mental health. Cyberpsychol Behav Soc Netw 17(10):652–657, 2014 25192305

Park SK, Kim JY, Cho CB: Prevalence of internet addiction and correlations with family factors among South Korean adolescents. Adolescence 43(172):895–909, 2008 19149152

Paulus FW, Ohmann S, von Gontard A, Popow C: Internet gaming disorder in children and adolescents: a systematic review. Dev Med Child Neurol 60(7):645–659, 2018 29633243

Shead S: Instagram and Snapchat were ranked the worst apps for children's mental health. Business Insider, May 19, 2017. Available at: https://www.businessinsider.com/instagram-and-snapchat-ranked-worsrt-childrens-mental-health-2017-5. Accessed March 2021.

Shek DTL, Tang VMY, Lo CY: Evaluation of an internet addiction treatment program for Chinese adolescents in Hong Kong. Adolescence 44(174):359–373, 2009 19764272

Sigman A: Virtually addicted: why general practice must now confront screen dependency. Br J Gen Pract 64(629):610–611, 2014 25452511

Song J, Park JH, Han DH, et al: Comparative study of the effects of bupropion and escitalopram on Internet gaming disorder. Psychiatry Clin Neurosci 70(11):527–535, 2016 27487975

Weinstein A, Livny A, Weizman A: New developments in brain research of internet and gaming disorder. Neurosci Biobehav Rev 75(April):314–330, 2017 28193454

Widyanto L, Griffiths M: 'Internet addiction': a critical review. Int J Ment Health Addict 4(1):31–51, 2006

World Health Organization: International Classification of Diseases and Related Health Problems, 11th Revision. Geneva, World Health Organization, 2019

Yen J-Y, Ko C-H, Yen C-F, et al: The comorbid psychiatric symptoms of internet addiction: attention deficit and hyperactivity disorder (ADHD), depression, social phobia, and hostility. J Adolesc Health 41(1):93–98, 2007 17577539

Young KS: Cognitive behavior therapy with internet addicts: treatment outcomes and implications. Cyberpsychol Behav 10(5):671–679, 2007 17927535

Zajac K, Ginley MK, Chang R, Petry NM: Treatments for internet gaming disorder and internet addiction: a systematic review. Psychol Addict Behav 31(8):979–994, 2017 28921996

CHAPTER NINE

Special Considerations for Older Adults

Seyed Parham Khalili, M.D., MAPP

> In the midst of winter, I found there was, within me, an invincible summer. For it says that no matter how hard the world pushes against me, within me, there's something stronger, something better, pushing right back.
>
> *Albert Camus (1970)*

Culture, Psychology, and Practice: Centuries in the Making

Over the past 200 years, steady advancements in technology have increasingly shaped the professional and personal lives of generations of adults. Early work in the 19th century focused particularly on the mechanics of calculating machines and steam-powered technology. Pioneers in the early to mid-20th century furthered these efforts, leading to pivotal developments such as the Turing machine, the Electronic Numerical Integrator and Calculator, the UNIVAC computer for business and governmental applications, computing languages, and progressively more sophisticated microchips. Further advancements in the second half of the 20th century led to additional hardware inventions such as Ethernet, commercially available business computers in the 1970s, the introduction of personal computing to American households through companies such as Sears and Roebuck in the 1980s, and HyperText Markup Language (better known as HTML) in 1990, eventually leading to the development of the World Wide Web. This, in turn, led to immersive gaming programs and sophisticated search engines such as Google in the late 1990s. Subsequent progress in the 21st century has ushered in a steady string of improvements in computing power, video-sharing services, social networking applications (apps), and immensely capable smartphones and tablet devices.

Throughout this whirlwind period of scientific innovation, different generations have had dramatically different experiences of living in a technologically minded, ever-changing world. Although much of the current news focuses on one particular generation—the Baby Boomers (born between 1946 and 1964)—other older adults, defined here as individuals age 60 and older, may belong to other cohorts and have also lived through an unprecedented period of advancement. In regard to specific cohorts during the past 138 years or so, older adults may be part of the Silent Generation (born between 1928 and 1945), the Greatest Generation (born between 1910 and 1927), the Interbellum Generation (born between 1901 and 1909), and even possibly the Lost Generation (born between 1883 and 1900). In comparison with Generation X (born between 1965 and 1980), Millenials (born between 1981 and 1996), and Generation Z (born in 1997 and later), the experiences of older adults could differ in myriad ways.

In general, these cohorts of older adults were significantly older than the younger generations when they were first introduced to personal computing, the internet, and other now ubiquitous forms of technological progress (Table 9–1). On first impression, this might suggest that older adults could be unlikely to integrate technology into their lives and that this would lead to a "digital divide" between "digital immigrants" (older adults) and "digital natives" (younger persons) (Nash 2019). Mass media and popular culture have often latched onto this notion, condoning if not promoting the stereotype of a technologically illiterate older person who is fearful of and willfully resistant to change. Fortunately, catalyzed by well-known demographic trends suggesting a near-doubling in the number of adults older than 65 years between 2020 and 2040, a multitude of researchers, clinicians, policymakers, and others are actively exploring different aspects of the interface between technology and aging (Administration for Community Living 2018). This evolving understanding about the role of technology in the lives of older adults, both in terms of positive changes and the risk for pathological pat-

TABLE 9–1. Selected milestones in technological innovation and median age by generation

Selected milestone (year)	Generation with respect to median age*				
	Generation Z	Millenials	Generation X	Baby Boomers	Silent Generation
IBM releases its first personal computer, nicknamed "Acorn" (1981)	Not yet born	Not yet born	8 years old	26 years old	46 years old
European Organization for Nuclear Research introduces the World Wide Web to the public (1991)	Not yet born	Not yet born	18 years old	36 years old	56 years old
Google developed at Stanford University (1996)	Not yet born	7 years old	23 years old	41 years old	61 years old
YouTube developed (2005)	0 years old	16 years old	32 years old	50 years old	70 years old
iPhone released (2007)	2 years old	18 years old	34 years old	52 years old	72 years old
iPad and Instagram released (2010)	5 years old	21 years old	37 years old	55 years old	75 years old
Facebook reaches 1 billion users (2012)	7 years old	23 years old	39 years old	57 years old	77 years old
Amazon Alexa released (2014)	9 years old	25 years old	41 years old	59 years old	79 years old
TikTok released (2016)	11 years old	27 years old	43 years old	61 years old	81 years old

*Approximate median birth year for each generation listed: Silent, 1935; Baby Boomers, 1955; Generation X, 1973; Millenials, 1989; Generation Z, 2005.

terns of use and other potential harms, is briefly discussed in the sections to follow.

Demographics and General Attitudes Toward Technology

At face value, many older adults appear to reside in somewhat similar regions and communities. Fifty-one percent of adults older than age 65 lived in just one of nine states in 2017, with 59% of community-dwelling adults reporting living with a spouse and relatively few living in long-term care facilities (Administration for Community Living 2018). There is, however, more variation in education level. Data from 2018 estimated that although at least 29% of adults over the age of 65 had obtained a bachelor's degree or higher, the percentage of people in this group who had completed high school differed by factors such as race/ethnicity, which ranged from 91% of non-Hispanic whites to 57% of Hispanics (Administration for Community Living 2018). Despite these educational differences, many older adults live with similar and substantial financial constraints. Nearly 90% of older adults receive Social Security payments, and these represent almost all of the monthly income for 21% of married and 45% of unmarried adults over the age of 65 (U.S. Social Security Administration 2016). According to U.S. Census data for 2017, the median income for survey respondents age 65 and older was $24,224, with 9.2% living below the poverty level. Moreover, 4.9% of survey respondents were categorized as "near poor," and only 24% of individuals reported an annual income of $50,000 or more (Administration for Community Living 2018).

These findings may shed light on which cohorts of older adults are adopting and actively using technology. Analyses from the Pew Center highlight a stronger positive correlation between technology use and socioeconomic factors. These factors include household income (>$75,000 vs. <$30,000), bachelor's and other advanced degrees (vs. high school diplomas or less schooling), and access to broadband services at home (vs. those who must access the internet in public places) (Anderson and Perrin 2017). Further helping to transcend the stereotyped view of older adults as technological outsiders is growing research demonstrating the rapid adoption of technology among adults age 65 and older.

Specific findings from the Pew Center for the period 2013–2017 examined ownership of smartphones (59% of those ages 65–69, 49% of those 70–74, 35% of those 75–79, and 17% of those >80), tablet computers (32% of adults ≥65), and e-readers (19% of adults ≥65). Additional data suggest that many older individuals (>65 years) use the internet at least daily (76%) and participate on some form of social media platform (34%) (Anderson and Perrin 2017). Findings from the American Association of Retired Persons (AARP) echo these trends, noting that most adults between the ages of 50 and 69 years use mobile technology for communication and entertainment. The use of desktop computers is more common among those age 70 and older, and relatively fewer older adults in general use their devices to manage finances or medical care compared with other activities (Anderson 2017). Although these data intimate that older adults do engage with technology, the impact of other demographic factors and older adults' views regarding technology are under continued investigation.

Research exploring older adults' perceptions about technology has provided insight. Some studies have found that older adults are more likely to adopt and use technology if the value and relevance to their personal lives are clear and outweigh perceived risk of harm (Fausset et al. 2013; Melenhorst et al. 2001). Work from the AARP also suggests that older adults think technology is positive for society as a whole and improves their quality of life by increasing access to entertainment, facilitating on-the-go activity, and improving communication with friends and family, although many worry about the privacy of personal and financial data, especially on social media sites (Anderson 2017). Among family units, another theme is that older adults value guidance from their children because this plays a significant role in influencing their likelihood to adopt newer technology (Fausset et al. 2013).

Although older persons are often grouped together based on age criteria, the cohort of adults age 65 and older encompasses people from different cultures, socioeconomic and educational backgrounds, religious and spiritual traditions, sexual preferences, gender identities, and life experiences. More research is needed to better understand how different older adults experience technology and which aspects of this relationship may be improved. We explore several themes in the existing literature on obstacles to using technology in the following sections.

Unique Issues for Older Adults

Related to the possible chasm mentioned earlier between digital natives and digital immigrants are the notions of "digital literacy" and "digital preparedness." *Digital preparedness* is generally interpreted as comfort level and confidence in one's ability to use technology, whereas *digital literacy* is defined as "the ability to use information and communication technologies to find, evaluate, create, and communicate information, requiring both cognitive and technical skills" (American Library Association 2020). These skill sets may be less sophisticated among some older adults. For example, findings by the AARP suggest that despite sometimes reporting a lack of trust in companies and organizations to protect their data, relatively few older adults take proactive steps to secure their information, even with respect to using passcodes or newer features such as two-factor identification (Anderson 2017).

Differences such as these could be due to physical problems, such as visual impairment or decreased fine motor control, or to issues related to experience and training. A larger proportion of older adults report a need for assistance when obtaining and using a new electronic device (Anderson and Perrin 2017). Moreover, those who have begun using at least one type of technology are more likely to adopt additional types moving forward, thereby also suggesting that a higher degree of familiarity and confidence with technology imbues a type of capital that may widen disparities between earlier adopters and later entrants (Anderson and Perrin 2017).

In addition to comfort and cumulative experience with technology, several types of psychological phenomena may also affect older adults differently. Social media platforms have been hypothesized to specifically arrange data and facilitate selected social endorsements that may then trigger decision heuristics, although the role of factors such as age and cognitive health is still unclear (Messing and Westwood 2012). Similarly, recent work has examined the phenomenon of "fake news" dissemination, defined here as "knowingly false or misleading content." Preliminary work suggests that although sharing this kind of content is uncommon overall, older adults may be significantly more likely to share it, even when controlling for variables such as political ideology and education level (Guess et al. 2019). This may be due to various contextual and psychological mechanisms.

One possible explanation includes the "illusion of truth" effect, where repetition bolsters belief in a false claim, possibly related to decreased recollection of the claim's original context (Skurnik et al. 2005). Another possible contributory factor may include the concept of the "continued influence effect of misinformation," which among older adults may be more pronounced and require more detailed counter information and reinforcement to overcome (Swire et al. 2017). The net effect of these phenomena and others in any given person or across the diverse cohort of older adults remains unclear and worthy of future research.

Addiction vs. Nonpathological Use

Before discussing some of the benefits of technology for older adults, it is helpful to identify several potential harms that may be unique to the geriatric population. As mentioned, certain older adults may face challenges in adopting technology and find themselves excluded from one or several aspects of modern life. Others may be at risk for financial exploitation and other predatory behavior perpetrated digitally. In some situations, older adults may even develop a pathological relationship to the technology itself or experience exacerbations of other behavioral- and substance-related disorders through their use of technology. In this section, we review several aspects of these interrelated phenomena.

Financial Scams and Mistreatment

Unfortunately, as increasing numbers of older adults have embraced technology and engaged in online activity, a myriad of financial scams have targeted them. Financial fraud and scams are now sadly a commonplace occurrence, on the order of billions of dollars annually. There is striking evidence that each year approximately 1 in 18 community-dwelling older adults falls victim to a scam (Burnes et al. 2017). The National Council on Aging has outlined 10 of the most common scams described by the FBI and other law enforcement and social service agencies. Often focusing on issues of particular interest to older adults, these scams may include health care and prescription medications, housing and retirement programs, investments and lotteries, charities seeking assistance, telemarketing scams, funeral and cemetery scams, and other types of fraud (National Council on Aging 2019). The perpetrator often poses as a family member, friend, or even a stranger in need. Although several of these scams are carried out by telephone, many are executed online, for example, through email/phishing scams and fraudulent websites that often appear legitimate at first glance.

The startling estimates of financial crimes against older adults may in fact still underestimate the true prevalence of the issue. Particularly susceptible older adults, such as those with a neurocognitive disorder, have been underrepresented in published analyses to date. This is particularly troubling given data suggesting that structural brain changes in older adults, especially in regions essential for socioemotional function, may be closely linked to risk for financial exploitation (Spreng et al. 2017). Perpetrators may be counting on these types of vulnerabilities, targeting older adults with the hope that they will be less vigilant about banking or data protection practices, more sympathetic to requests for assistance, impaired in cognition or general health, and socially isolated or lonely. Older adults may also be less likely than younger adults to report these incidents. Consequently, these crimes can be devastating for older adults and their families, both financially and psychologically. Of note, in situations in which the perpetrator is someone for whom the older adult would have an *expectation of trust*, for example, a family member or caregiver, this type of criminal activity could also be categorized as a form of financial elder mistreatment (elder abuse). Although these types of behaviors are distinct from the notion of a technological addiction, they are not exclusive, thereby making awareness of financial fraud essential among both older adults and their health care providers.

Defining Pathological Technology Use

Distinguishing between healthy and pathological use of technology is a challenging endeavor. Clinicians must consider many potential medical, psychiatric, and socioeconomic confounders that may be unique among a geriatric population. Before delving deeper, let us begin with a basic description of the dividing line between *addiction* and *nonpathological use*, drawing on overlapping concepts in psychiatry and geriatric medicine.

Although specific diagnostic criteria are reviewed in other sections, problematic internet use (PIU), or internet addiction (IA), is reviewed here as it pertains to older populations. PIU is an umbrella term that may include various specific online behaviors that have become maladaptive. Given that the study of technological addictions is a relatively new endeavor without a universal set of criteria, the epidemiology of PIU remains unclear. Across even technologically advanced societies, estimates of prevalence range from 1% to 36.7% (Ko et al. 2012). Here PIU could include many behaviors, such as general internet use and social networking, gaming, shopping and auction participation, gambling, pornography, and other activities. A recent two-site survey across the United States and South Africa suggested that online activities appeared to differ across age, with subgroup analysis of PIU among adults age 55 and older suggesting a stronger association with general internet surfing, "time wasters," and media-streaming services in particular (Ioannidis et al. 2018).

Deciding whether the behavior represents a technological addiction can be difficult, given the ongoing work clarifying specific diagnostic criteria. Compatible with both DSM-5 (American Psychiatric Association 2013) and geriatric approaches to diagnosis, however, a focus on function and functional trajectories may be a useful initial frame of reference for older adults. Specifically, this includes considering how the behavior may be affecting the person's day-to-day activity and vocational, interpersonal, and societal participation. Extrapolating from psychiatric and psychological assessments of substance-related and behavioral addictions (e.g., gambling disorder), additional features suggestive of pathological use of technology may include preoccupation with the activity, the need to spend significant and progressively more time on the activity, euphoria or a reduction in dysphoria with participation in the activity, withdrawal-like symptoms when reducing or ceasing the activity, a sense of loss of control and ongoing use despite harm to self, and other negative consequences.

It is also helpful to discuss one phenomenon that is receiving more attention in studies of older adults—social media use—with the caveat that this behavior is also explored in more detail in Chapter 6. Social media platforms provide many older adults, particularly those limited by physical and financial constraints, with an opportunity to engage with a community beyond the confines of their homes. Simultaneously, as some preliminary work has found, both problematic social media use and depression may be highly correlated with higher perceived social isolation. This suggests that the way social media is used is essential when assessing whether it is helpful or inadvertently harmful (Meshi et al. 2020). In the absence of specific DSM-5 criteria for this condition, the onus of diagnosis falls on clinicians, who are charged with performing a detailed physical and psychiatric assessment to discern whether the technological behavior is causing harm.

Similarly, among comprehensive geriatric assessments (described later), a focus on functional status may draw on a review of activities of daily living, instrumental activities of daily living, vocational and societal participation, interpersonal relationships and caregiving (received or provided), and phenotypic geriatric syndromes such as frailty, cognitive impairment, and other biopsychosocial phenomena. This congruence between disciplines highlights a sort of shared language that is not only employable during holistic, person-centered assessments of individuals but also vital to our growing understanding of technological addictions among older adults. In this vein, practitioners, patients, and families are afforded a more generous toolkit with which to approach the problem and devise solutions.

Positive Aspects

Much of the discussion thus far has centered on potential challenges and pitfalls that older adults may face. However, much remains to be said regarding the numerous positive aspects of technology for a geriatric population. Accessible, thoughtfully designed devices and software can broaden the reach and depth of social, medical, and economic initiatives aimed at improving quality of life for older adults. Selected innovative work by a diverse group of researchers and organizations is described further to provide a few examples of potential benefits.

Reducing Loneliness and Social Isolation

Aptly described as "the new geriatric giants," social isolation and loneliness pose serious short- and long-term risks for older adults in a wide variety of community and clinical settings (Freedman and Nicolle 2020). *Social isola-*

tion commonly refers to an absence of social connections, whereas *loneliness* refers to the subjective feeling of being alone (Gardiner et al. 2018). Adverse consequences can include physical and psychological morbidity, increased mortality, accelerated functional decline, higher avoidable health care utilization and costs, heightened risk for elder mistreatment, and decreased self-reported quality of life. Preliminarily, it appears less likely that social isolation and loneliness would be products of technology and PIU, as they might be among younger adults struggling with social media, for example. Rather, among older adults it may be that risk factors for isolation and loneliness may themselves be obstacles to healthy technology use, although technology may be a potent tool with which to augment socialization and combat the consequences of loneliness.

Information and communication technologies, although a heterogeneous group of devices and approaches, have been viewed as possible interventions. Some examples include telephone/video software, including peer support programs and social media sites, video games, personal robotics, telemedicine, and three-dimensional virtual environments. Unfortunately, findings to date have been mixed. One recent randomized controlled trial of a computer system specifically designed for older adults, called the Personal Reminder Information and Social Management (PRISM) system, found an increase in measurements of social connectivity and self-efficacy and less reported loneliness (Czaja et al. 2018). However, a recent systematic review of somewhat similar technology suggested nonsignificant or even negative effects on loneliness, equivocal effects on self-efficacy or self-esteem, and perhaps only short-term benefits for social connectedness and activity participation (Chen and Schulz 2016).

Technological interventions for social isolation and loneliness are probably also more likely to be effective if they pay heed to several key concepts from the broader literature. These may include adaptability (i.e., being applicable to the diverse needs of older adults who may live in significantly different settings with various levels of autonomy and needs), a community development approach (i.e., meaningfully including older adults in the planning and implementation states of the interventions), and productive engagement (i.e., prioritizing interventions that facilitate active involvement by the user as opposed to passive consumption) (Gardiner et al. 2018). Future work might help address some of the limitations of earlier studies on social interventions or "social prescribing" that were limited in scope or lacked robust methodologies, as well as pay greater attention to particularly vulnerable yet underrepresented populations, such as cognitively impaired persons.

Providing Education

Many information and communication technologies offer educational resources to a wide audience of older adults who may otherwise lack access. Fortunately, many reputable institutions and organizations have programs with content specifically designed for older adults. The AARP offers educational programs and resources online. Another source of high-quality education and resources is an organization called Older Adults Technology Services. Its flagship program, Senior Planet, has a range of training courses on different types of technology through online and community-based programming. Finally, the U.S. Department of Aging website offers a multitude of resources for health, legal, education, and retirement issues, including links to local resources that may be of service.

Improving Health and Promoting "Aging in Place"

The role of technology in improving health and helping older adults continue living at home and avoid institutionalization ("aging in place") is an active area of inquiry and innovation. Telemedicine services have continued to grow throughout the COVID-19 pandemic, offering expanded access to primary and specialty providers for older adults who may otherwise face barriers to receiving care safely in traditional health care settings. Even prior to the pandemic, these obstacles included geographical provider shortages, mobility, and cost, to name just a few. According to the AARP, among adults older than 60 years, laptop computers are the most popular type of device for health-related activities (34% use them to receive and manage medical care and 43% use them for health information), with smartphones and tablets being used less often for these purposes (Anderson 2017).

In other published work, older adults expressed interest in patient portals for access to their electronic medical records and care coordination and a particular desire for apps/programs that can facilitate self-awareness about health behaviors, provide coaching and guidance, and help prevent overall functional decline (Cabrita et al. 2019; Portz et al. 2019). With support from family, friends, and caregivers, these types of services could allow older adults to remain in their homes and communities and delay or prevent a potentially undesired transition to a long-term care facility, not only reducing health care expenditures but also optimizing quality of life, social connections, and autonomy.

Treatment

There is growing interest in how to best tailor general medical and mental health services to the needs of older adults. However, there is as yet a paucity of published comparative effectiveness research on specific treatments for technological and behavioral addictions, making best practices unclear. Treatments for different technological and behavioral addictions are described elsewhere in their respective chapters of this book and would also be applicable to older adults. Similarly, treatment for co-occurring psychiatric disorders would be necessary and may serve both therapeutic and diagnostic purposes because some aspects of the addiction-like behavior may potentially improve. From a health care systems perspective, however, several overarching principles can be extrapolated from the larger spheres of primary care, geriatrics, and psychiatry. Key aspects of the patient-centered medical home and behavioral health home models for care may be applied to the treatment approach for technological addictions.

A patient-centered medical home is a concept initially developed in the 1960s by clinicians and policymakers interested in prioritizing the role of patients in health care delivery. It was further expanded to encompass high-quality, empathic, patient-centered care using evidence-based practices. A behavioral health home is often defined as a behavioral health agency that serves as the centerpiece in care delivery and coordination for individuals with mental health and substance use disorders. The ideal behavioral health home personifies four principles of effective care within a chronic-care model: person-centered care, population-based care, data-driven care, and evidence-based care (Center for Integrated Health Solutions 2012).

Person-centered care suggests that all care should be based on the person's preferences, needs, and values and frequently leverages self-management support to facilitate collaborative decision-making between patients and providers. *Population-based care* encapsulates a multitude of approaches for evaluating, tracking, and improving the health of an entire population through case management. This includes tools for proactively identifying patient needs and effectively coordinating care delivery. *Data-driven care* means that validated assessment tools are used to collect clinical data that are then organized and reviewed for the purposes of fine-tuning care. Finally, *evidence-based care* consists of combining clinical expertise with the best available published evidence to guide treatment decisions for not only acute care needs but also prevention, health promotion, and health education.

Considering that older adults are well known to be more likely to experience multimorbidity, physical limitations, financial stressors, and progressive needs for caregiving as they age, the comprehensive and data-driven strategic approach of a behavioral health home is also a logical system within which to incorporate assessments and treatments for technological/behavioral addictions. More information about the specific processes and strategies for behavioral health homes can be found on the Substance Abuse and Mental Health Services Administration and U.S. Health Resources and Services Administration websites.

Special Considerations

Regarding assessments for both the substance-related and technological/behavioral addictions, clinical assessments of older adults are more likely to be informative and accurate when certain factors are considered and explored. Older adults are not only more likely to experience medical issues related to individual organs or biological systems but also more likely to experience multimorbidity, as noted earlier. Multimorbidity, either alone or in conjunction with other socioeconomic and psychological factors, can culminate in geriatric syndromes. These syndromes represent phenotypic states that can have significant implications for morbidity, mortality, and daily functioning. As such, an evaluation for geriatric syndromes represents a major goal of any comprehensive geriatric assessment, which is the systematic evaluation of medical, psychological, and social health and functioning.

In practice, the differential diagnosis for a constellation of historical and clinical data may be both broad and nuanced among older adults, particularly when compared with generally healthy younger adults. Individual disease processes and geriatric syndromes can differ in their presentations compared with "textbook" descriptions. In some cases, physical findings may be very subtle, or the presentation may differ altogether, with symptoms that are rarely seen in younger persons. Furthermore, the lived experience of the older adult, including cultural norms, relationship to health and health care systems, prior trauma, and other variables, may uniquely influence the assessment and presentation. Clinicians may employ a number of strategies to help overcome some of these inherent challenges when assessing a technological behavioral pattern.

Specifically, when evaluating an older adult for issues pertaining to use of technology and its impact, clinicians may wish to invest additional time on several components of the history and physical assessment. With respect to obtaining a history, although no diagnostic criteria have been universally agreed upon for most types of technological or behavioral addictions, it is nonetheless helpful to revisit the conceptual framework described earlier during the discussion of pathological technology use. In addition to speaking with the patient, clinicians can request permission to include other persons involved in the patient's life. Interviewing family members, close friends, caregivers, care recipients, and other individuals close to the older adult is often instrumental. This information can clarify the impact of the technology use over time and in different settings or contexts.

The clinician can specifically probe for signs that the relationship between the person and the technology is marked by issues such as a loss of control over the behavior, euphoria experienced during the behavior, dysphoria during reduction or cessation of the behavior, compulsion to continue the behavior despite negative consequences, and, in harmony with a geriatric medicine approach, a reasonable estimation that the behavior is compromising overall functional status in terms of usual activity, important relationships, and long-held values and preferences. This process might be contentious, because patients and others involved in their lives may differ in opinion regarding the patient's relationship to technology. Furthermore, the diagnosis or answer may not be readily apparent on first appraisal and may require repeat assessments over time, ideally in a setting that is conducive to establishing trust and continuity of care between the clinician and the older adult.

Tangential to the usual data-gathering process employed while interviewing patients and sources of collateral information about the patients' behaviors, it may be useful to also screen for any financial exploitation that might be present. Sometimes, this information may arise organically from the review of the patient's actions and perceived associated outcomes. However, sometimes patients and others in their lives may be hesitant to disclose instances of financial mistreatment out of embarrassment, fear of loss of autonomy over finances and other decisions, or even culpability for the caregiver, friend, or family member. Nonetheless, attempting to include these types of questions into the assessment affords the clinician an additional opportunity to evaluate for technology-related issues caused by a physical or cognitive impairment, technological addictions such as PIU, signs of elder mistreatment, or a separate type of financial fraud.

Given findings that associate some patterns of technology use and technological addictions with other mental health disorders, assessment of an older adult's mental health is essential. This includes an initial screening followed by a more comprehensive evaluation when warranted. A careful interview may provide context with respect to prior illness and treatment experiences, ongoing risk factors, potential co-occurring psychiatric diagnoses, and available support systems. Specific screening for depression, anxiety, and cognitive impairment is a good first step, using whichever specific instruments are most feasible in the respective practice setting. Although limited, literature particular to PIU among middle-age and older adults suggests a stronger correlation with several conditions, relative to younger adults. Specifically, major depressive disorder, general anxiety disorder, and OCD have been identified as conditions to be considered by clinicians during assessment (Ioannidis et al. 2018). For individuals who already carry one or more other psychiatric diagnoses, it may be helpful to elucidate the trajectory of these conditions, particularly with respect to the effect of the technological behavior and how treatment approaches may be coordinated.

In addition to a thorough interview, a careful physical examination can serve multiple functions. It can reveal medical issues that may be contributing to problematic use of technology or may separately need attention. Moreover, the examination can highlight clusters of findings that may meet criteria for a geriatric syndrome, such as frailty, that imparts additional information about the likely functional trajectory of that person over time. In addition, a meticulous examination can often help rule out certain confounders that may lead to a false-positive initial impression of a behavioral or psychiatric diagnosis. Finally, discernment of physical and cognitive limitations can provide an opportunity to identify potential interventions that may assist the older adult in safely and productively becoming more engaged in care and subsequently using technology productively. Specific suggestions are provided in Table 9–2 and can be initially performed in an office-based or even telemedicine-based encounter by a wide range of clinicians, with referral for follow-up testing in specialty clinics if appropriate.

KEY POINTS

- Older adults are more likely to adopt new technology when they perceive its value and have access to assistance when they encounter obstacles.

- Older adults face unique challenges associated with different degrees of digital literacy and digital preparedness, often along with aging-related multimorbidity and cognitive changes.

- Potential harms associated with technology use among older adults may include financial exploitation and addiction to technology.

- Technology offers older adults many potential benefits across the domains of education, health, and self-efficacy, with opportunities for greater engagement in a global society.

- Although best practices in technological addiction treatments are not yet clear, older adults will likely benefit from the same approaches as younger adults, particularly in a behavioral health home model for care delivery.

TABLE 9–2. Clinical considerations during assessment

System	Examination	Rationale
Visual	Office-based vision screening	May preclude use of visual technology or contribute to incorrect use, confusion/delirium, distress, increased vulnerability to online scams
	Referral for ophthalmological or optometric assessment	Potentially treatable with refractive lenses or other interventions
Auditory	Office-based hearing screening	Impairment in hearing may preclude use of auditory technology, contribute to incorrect use, confusion/delirium, distress, vulnerability to telephone scams
	Referral to audiology for formal testing	Potentially treatable with hearing aids or other interventions
Musculoskeletal and neurological	Level of alertness, cranial nerve examination, range of motion and signs of arthropathy (especially upper extremities), strength, muscle tone, dexterity and fine motor control (especially upper extremities), gait and balance	May inhibit use of computers and other devices; some limitations potentially treatable with prosthetics or device modifications
	Cognitive testing with a formal instrument such as a Montreal Cognitive Assessment or Mini-Mental Status Exam	Neurodegenerative conditions can include different types of cognitive impairment and psychological and perceptual changes that may inhibit effective use of technology and increase susceptibility to financial scams
	Additional neurocognitive testing pending screening and clinical findings	
	Financial capacity assessment by an experienced clinician if needed	

TABLE 9–2. Clinical considerations during assessment *(continued)*

System	Examination	Rationale
Psychiatric	Mental status examination	Differential diagnosis of a technological-behavioral addiction can include another psychiatric condition
	Depression screening using formal instrument such as the Patient Health Questionnaire–9, Geriatric Depression Scale, or other tool	Provides an opportunity to simultaneously treat co-occurring conditions in a behavioral health home model of care
	Anxiety screening using General Anxiety Disorder–7 or another tool	
	Screening for substance use disorders and other conditions if applicable	

Practice Questions

1. An 82-year-old man with hypertension and chronic pain related to osteo-arthritis presents to your clinic with his daughter for assessment of "a mood problem." He is withdrawn and minimally engaged during the interview. He also provides permission for his daughter to participate in his assessment, and she reports that he spends most of the day in front of the computer playing games and browsing the internet.

   Which of the following statements is most likely to suggest a possible pathological use of technology?

   A. He visits the same websites every day.
   B. He reports feeling depressed most days of the week.
   C. He has difficulty seeing the computer screen and using a mouse effectively.
   D. He reports difficulty with controlling how much time he spends online and with cutting down his use despite a desire to do so.
   E. He made several expensive purchases online in the past month.

   Answer: D.

   Core features of pathological technology use include a loss of control over the behavior and difficulty reducing use despite a desire to do so. The other answer options may represent the patient's preferences (A); co-occurring symptoms that may or may not be related to a technological addiction (B); physical challenges in using technology, such as with vision or fine motor control (C); and choices that may or may not be prudent but are not pathognomonic for a disorder in and of themselves (E).

2. Which of the following statements about older adults and technology is most accurate based on recent patterns and observations?

   A. Older adults rarely use technology, especially after age 70.
   B. Older adults tend not to worry about online privacy and banking.
   C. Because they have been around technology longer, older adults are more skillful users.
   D. More than one-third of adults older than 65 engage in some form of social media.
   E. Financial fraud has become rare among older adults due to online protections.

Answer: D.

Growing numbers of older adults are participating in various applications and online services, including social media. Although patterns in technology use may vary with age, significant numbers of adults older than 70 years engage with technology (A), many older adults report worrying about loss of their data online (B), some older adults struggle with digital literacy and digital preparedness, in part because they were introduced to technology later in life in comparison with younger users (C), and financial fraud has become a commonplace occurrence (E), with new inroads online and through other digital media.

3. A 76-year-old woman with diabetes, dyslipidemia, and generalized anxiety disorder presents for routine follow-up accompanied by her full-time caregiver and brings with her a tablet device that she recently purchased. She excitedly demonstrates how she uses the tablet and frequently scrolls through a social media site during the encounter, struggling to maintain her focus on the interview and assessment.

   Which of the following approaches may be most helpful in exploring the possibility of pathological use of the technology?

   A. Reviewing the social media site to see if her posts receive significant numbers of "likes" and positive feedback
   B. Counting the number of times she uses the device during the encounter
   C. With her permission, discussing her pattern of use of the device with her caregiver, including questions about changes in her interpersonal relationships, time spent on other activities that are important to her, and possible effects on her overall daily functioning
   D. Evaluating how skillfully she can use the device to perform internet searches, open programs, and perform other functions
   E. Comparing her level of skill using the device with that of other patients around her age who also attend your clinic

Answer: C.

Other core features of pathological technology use include negative effects on relationships, vocation, and activities that are meaningful to the affected person. With permission from the patient, the clinician could speak to the caregiver to probe for these possibilities. The other options do not by themselves point to pathological use—whether she is popular on social media (A), uses the device frequently (B), is skillful in using the device (D), or has more or less skill with the device than her peers (E).

Resources for Clinicians, Patients, and Families

American Association of Retired Persons (https://aarp.org)
Older Adults Technology Services (https://oats.org/#)
U.S. Department of Health and Human Services (www.hhs.gov/aging)
U.S. Department on Aging Eldercare Locator (https://eldercare.acl.gov/Public/Index.aspx)

References

Administration for Community Living: 2018 Profile of Older Americans. Washington, DC, Administration for Community Living, 2018. Available at: https://acl.gov/sites/default/files/Aging and Disability in America/2018OlderAmericansProfile.pdf

American Library Association: Digital Literacy. ALA.org, 2020. Available at: https://literacy.ala.org/digital-literacy. Accessed April 4, 2020.

American Psychiatric Association: Diagnostic and Statistical Manual of Mental Disorders, 5th Edition. Arlington, VA, American Psychiatric Association, 2013

Anderson GO: Technology Use and Attitudes Among Mid-Life and Older Americans. Washington, DC, American Association of Retired Persons, 2017. Available at: https://www.aarp.org/content/dam/aarp/research/surveys_statistics/technology/info-2018/atom-nov-2017-tech-module.doi.10.26419%252Fres.00210.001.pdf. Accessed March 21, 2020.

Anderson M, Perrin A: Tech adoption climbs among older adults. Pew Research Center: Internet and Tech, May 17, 2017. Available at: https://www.pewresearch.org/internet/2017/05/17/tech-adoption-climbs-among-older-adults. Accessed February 8, 2020.

Burnes D, Henderson CR Jr, Sheppard C, et al: Prevalence of financial fraud and scams among older adults in the United States: a systematic review and meta-analysis. Am J Public Health 107(8):e13–e21, 2017 28640686

Cabrita M, Tabak M, Vollenbroek-Hutten MM: Older adults' attitudes toward ambulatory technology to support monitoring and coaching of healthy behaviors: qualitative study. JMIR Aging 2(1):e10476, 2019 31518252

Camus A: Return to Tipasa, in Lyrical and Critical Essays. Edited by Thody P. New York, Vintage Books, 1970

Center for Integrated Health Solutions: Behavioral Health Homes for People With Mental Health and Substance Use Conditions: The Core Clinical Features.

Washington, DC, Substance Abuse and Mental Health Services Administration–Health Resources and Services Administration, 2012

Chen YR, Schulz PJ: The effect of information communication technology interventions on reducing social isolation in the elderly: a systematic review. J Med Internet Res 18(1):e18, 2016 26822073

Czaja SJ, Boot WR, Charness N, et al: Improving social support for older adults through technology: findings from the PRISM randomized controlled trial. Gerontologist 58(3):467–477, 2018 28201730

Fausset CB, Harvey L, Farmer S, Fain B: Older adults' perceptions and use of technology: a novel approach, in Universal Access in Human-Computer Interaction: User and Context Diversity. Edited by Stephanidis C. Berlin, Springer, 2013, pp 51–58

Freedman A, Nicolle J: Social isolation and loneliness: the new geriatric giants: approach for primary care. Can Fam Physician 66(3):176–182, 2020 32165464

Gardiner C, Geldenhuys G, Gott M: Interventions to reduce social isolation and loneliness among older people: an integrative review. Health Soc Care Community 26(2):147–157, 2018 27413007

Guess A, Nagler J, Tucker J: Less than you think: prevalence and predictors of fake news dissemination on Facebook. Sci Adv 5(1):eaau4586, 2019 30662946

Ioannidis K, Treder MS, Chamberlain SR, et al: Problematic internet use as an age-related multifaceted problem: evidence from a two-site survey. Addict Behav 81:157–166, 2018 29459201

Ko CH, Yen JY, Yen CF, et al: The association between internet addiction and psychiatric disorder: a review of the literature. Eur Psychiatry 27(1):1–8, 2012 22153731

Melenhorst AS, Rogers W, Caylor E: The use of communication technologies by older adults: exploring the benefits from the user's perspective, in Proceedings of the Human Factors and Ergonomics Society 45th Annual Meeting, Minneapolis, MN, October 2001, pp 221–225

Meshi D, Cotten SR, Bender AR: Problematic social media use and perceived social isolation in older adults: a cross-sectional study. Gerontology 66(2):160–168, 2020 31522178

Messing S, Westwood SJ: Selective exposure in the age of social media: endorsements trump partisan source affiliation when selecting news online. Communic Res 41(8):1042–1063, 2012

Nash S: Older adults and technology: moving beyond the stereotypes. Stanford Center on Longevity, April 13, 2019. Available at: https://longevity.stanford.edu/older-adults-and-technology-moving-beyond-the-stereotypes. Accessed February 8, 2020.

National Council on Aging: Top 10 financial scams targeting seniors. NCOA.org, 2019. Available at: https://www.ncoa.org/economic-security/money-management/scams-security/top-10-scams-targeting-seniors. Accessed February 8, 2020.

Portz JD, Bayliss EA, Bull S, et al: Using the technology acceptance model to explore user experience, intent to use, and use behavior of a patient portal among older adults with multiple chronic conditions: descriptive qualitative study. J Med Internet Res 21(4):e11604, 2019 30958272

Skurnik I, Yoon C, Park D, Schwarz N: How warnings about false claims become recommendations. J Consum Res 31:713–724, 2005

Spreng RN, Cassidy BN, Darboh BS, et al: Financial exploitation is associated with structural and functional brain differences in healthy older adults. J Gerontol A Biol Sci Med Sci 72(10):1365–1368, 2017 28369260

Swire B, Ecker UKH, Lewandowsky S: The role of familiarity in correcting inaccurate information. J Exp Psychol Learn Mem Cogn 43(12):1948–1961, 2017 28504531

U.S. Social Security Administration: Fact sheet: Social Security. Washington, DC, Social Security Administration, 2016. Available at: https://www.ssa.gov/news/press/factsheets/basicfact-alt.pdf. Accessed February 8, 2020.

CHAPTER TEN

New and Emerging Addictive Technologies

Where Do We Go From Here?

Rafael Coira, M.D., J.D.

Unhappy man! Do you share my madness? Have you drunk also of the intoxicating draught? Hear me; let me reveal my tale, and you will dash the cup from your lips!

Mary Shelley, Frankenstein

You could potentially download [memories] into a new body or a robot body. The future is going to be weird.

Elon Musk

Culture, Psychology, and Practice

Transhumanism

They call it the "eyeborg" (Stix 2016). Neil Harbisson was born without something many of us take for granted: the ability to see color. As an artist, he was limited to painting in black and white (Brennan 2008), and as a musician, he was drawn to the piano with its black and white keys. However, Harbisson suffers from those limitations no longer, because he is no longer human. Neil Harbisson is a cyborg.

It may sound like science fiction, but it is fact. In 2004, a physician implanted a device, created by Harbisson, into his skull. The eyeborg allows him to *hear* colors. The device is fused with his occiput, and by passing vibrations into his skull, it allows him to perceive the colors to which he was once blind. His newfound abilities do not stop there; the eyeborg also allows him to see what others cannot. He can perceive infrared and ultraviolet colors; colors that are beyond the visible spectrum. Through an internet connection on his appendage, he can receive signals from space, videos, phone calls, and more (Cyborg Arts 2020).

Harbisson is a pioneer in a movement known as *transhumanism*. Whether seeking to overcome limitations or simply to reach new heights, transhumanists advocate for the use of technology to transcend the current human form and transition into a future species. The possibilities are limitless, and the current examples are surprisingly ubiquitous. In fact, according to Elon Musk, we are all cyborgs already. Musk, the founder of SpaceX and Tesla, believes that the smartphones in our hands are an extension of our human body; one that allows us to access all of the world's knowledge in an instant and much more. Taking this logic to the extreme, however, a caveman with a stone ax would then be considered a cyborg, eroding the utility of the term. Would permanently attaching the stone to his hand make it so? Where between our cave-dwelling roots and our spacefaring destiny does this transition from human to posthuman occur? Let us examine some other examples of today.

Take, for instance, Kevin Warwick and his Project Cyborg (Warwick et al. 2003). By implanting an electrode array into his median nerve, the noted engineer was able to control a robotic hand and a wheelchair on the other side of the Atlantic. With this technology he was further able to achieve extrasensory perception and, via electrodes implanted into his wife's peripheral nervous system, telepathy. What is perhaps most amazing about these experiments is that they are almost a quarter of a century old.

The examples of cyborgs are all mostly human with a bit of machine, but as the technological capabilities expand, we can expect that ratio to tip in the other direction. For example, it has long been a science fiction trope and a distant fantasy to upload the human brain into a computer or cloud, but some think we may be on the cusp of making that dream a reality. The 2045 Strategic Social Initiative (2045.com), founded by Russian billionaire Dmitry Itskov, describes its primary objective thus: "to create technologies enabling the transfer of [an] individual's personality to a more advanced non-biological carrier, and extending life, including to the point of immortality" (2045 Strategic Social Initiative 2020). Specifically, by 2045, Itskov's goal is for "substance-independent minds" to receive "new bodies with capacities far exceeding those of ordinary humans" (2045 Strategic Social Initiative 2020).

Itskov's iteration opens endless possibilities and, with them, endless addictive perils. Suddenly, for the right price, anything would be possible: a perfect body, an angelic voice, unassisted flight, instant knowledge, superintelligence, and the list goes on. If robotic body manufacturers are anything like smartphone producers, we could expect a new and improved model every year at escalating prices. However, a robotic shell does not need to be infused with human intelligence to be addictive. Artificial intelligence (AI) will be just as effective.

Artificial Intelligence

AI, perhaps the trendiest technology of our time, may also be one of the most difficult to delineate: a property attributable to the nebulous nature of intelligence itself. One measure of AI is the Turing test. Devised in the middle of the 20th century by British computer scientist Alan Turing, the test challenges human judges to distinguish a machine from a human based on printed conversation. If the human evaluator cannot reliably identify which dialogue came from the machine and which came from the human, the machine is deemed to have passed the test. Not infrequently, researchers or businesses garner considerable attention by claiming to have developed a machine that passes the Turing test, but such claims are generally met with skepticism and rebuttals. Many hold that the Turing test has never been passed. Perhaps more hold that it is a fool's errand in the first place.

The Turing test is beautiful in its breadth and simplicity. With a relatively limited—although debated—set of requirements, it lends itself to the breadth of subject matter that makes us human. It also emphasizes reason and wit rather than data storage and retrieval. Yet the test has many valid criticisms. One is that it tests whether a machine can be like a human rather than whether it is intelligent. *Intelligence*, it can be argued, is not exclusively human, nor are humans always intelligent. Is a machine not intelligent if it achieves some level of intelligence but not sufficient intelligence to eclipse that of a human? Which human should we compare a machine to? A similar detraction to the Turing test is that it can be considered a test of deception rather than intelligence. This point can be illustrated by the case of Eugene Goostman.

Eugene Goostman was not a man but, rather, a piece of software that purportedly passed the Turing test in 2014 (BBC News 2014). By pretending to be a 13-year-old Ukrainian boy, the chatbot was able to convince one-third of judges at the United Kingdom's Royal Society that it was human. In this context, grammatical errors and idiosyncrasies could be attributed to Goostman's age and foreign nationality. Perhaps if Goostman had devised the deceptive strategy itself, its creators would have an argument for having achieved human level intelligence; however, the plan was a product of the biological mind of its human programmers. Indeed, the mechanical responses in several published conversations between individuals and Goostman lead one to wonder how the judges might have been fooled in the first place. These and other detractions led some to believe that the Turing test is an unnecessary distraction from the real work of AI. Others suggest that the test is not a test at all but more of a principle or benchmark. Although the debate can easily be dismissed as a matter of semantics, what cannot be dismissed is the impact the field of AI is having and will continue to have on our lives. The field can be broken down into several overlapping subfields; let us examine a few to understand how they might have addictive potential.

Natural language processing (NLP) is a branch of AI that concerns itself with programming computers to understand humans in their natural language. Historically, in order to interact with computers, we have been limited to giving specific instructions—in essence, speaking *their* language or at best some intermediary. In contrast, the aim of NLP is for humans to interact meaningfully with computers by speaking in plain tongue. As is apparent to anyone who has had a conversation with Siri, Alexa, or Cortana, the field has made tremendous strides in recent years. What is likely also apparent is that these specific iterations of NLP are a far cry from the ability to carry on a conversation with the depth or breadth we generally expect from other humans (Garbade 2018).

Apple's Siri, Amazon's Alexa, and Microsoft's Cortana are well known examples of virtual assistants that rely on NLP to interact with their humans. These pieces of software can perform many tasks, such as tell you the weather, talk to you about movies or sporting events, play games, and, unsurprisingly, sell you things. Other technologies that harness NLP include translating, voice text messaging, and identifying related keywords on databases and search engines. Many NLP applications use the next aspect of AI: machine learning. Machine learning is the use of computer algorithms that self-improve through experience. More specifically, machine learning leverages computers' ability to determine probabilities. By feeding a computer a data set annotated with correct answers and allowing the algorithms to churn through that information repeatedly, the computer refines its ability to accurately predict the correct responses by rearranging the questions asked and the order in which they are asked (Harris 2018). So, for example, car company Tesla's autopilot system learns to identify stop signs by being fed countless images of objects that are and are not stop signs, keeping track of the images that indeed contain stop signs. Through countless repetition, the computer improves its ability to discriminate between them.

Machine learning can rely on several methods; the most accurate to date is the deep neural network, whose basic idea is to break information down into constituent chunks or "neurons" and allow the computer to analyze successive layers of thousands of neurons. The computer then determines the probability that the identified pattern represents the thing for which it has been designed to look (Harris 2018). One of the major drawbacks to this approach is the same problem that computers have always had: garbage in, garbage out. If the computer is given a data set that tells it that stop signs are three-sided and yellow, the computer may reliably misidentify yield signs as stop signs and ignore red octagonal signs, with potentially catastrophic results. That said, a human pupil would be similarly susceptible, although one would expect a human with a broader life experience and knowledge base to quickly figure out that he or she had been misled. The person might determine the correct meaning of a sign through the process of generalizing past experiences and applying them to the current situation. For example, although the person may not be familiar with traffic signs, he or she has learned in other contexts that red is the color often used to signify stop or danger. The extent to which computers can similarly question and correct their own programmers may improve as machine learning methods become increasingly more sophisticated.

Virtual Reality

In 1832, prolific inventor Charles Wheatstone developed the first stereoscope, a device that capitalizes on humans' binocular depth perception to create an immersive visual experience akin to, although distinct from, three-dimensional (3D) imaging. Variations of his device are still popular today. Stereoscopes deliver separate images of the same scene to each eye at slightly different perspectives, roughly the perspectives each eye would see if one were standing at the scene, leading to the illusion of 3D depth. Later renditions of Wheatstone's stereoscope include 1939's Viewmaster and 2014's Google Cardboard. Although cave drawings or even oral traditions could be considered simulations of reality, the stereoscope represents a particular leap forward in immersion noted as a major steppingstone along the path toward what would eventually be known as virtual reality or VR (Virtual Reality Society 2020).

Today, VR is relatively ubiquitous. This book is being written during the COVID-19 pandemic. For many in the United States, the first realization of the level of disruption COVID would have on society came when the National Basketball Association suddenly and dramatically suspended the 2020 season. On March 11, 2020, Utah Jazz player Rudy Gobert tested positive for the novel coronavirus, leading to a league-wide suspension of the season moments before tip-off of the Jazz-Thunder game (Aschburner 2020). Soon, no traditional major sports would be played—college basketball, hockey, soccer, the Olympics, auto racing, and so on—and in their place would be virtual versions of the real thing, with familiar athletes venturing into the unfamiliar realm of e-sports.

Determined to continue, NASCAR (2020) went virtual with the eNASCAR iRacing Pro Invitational Series. The series pitted NASCAR drivers against each other on virtual versions of the tracks on which they would have been racing if the series had not been suspended. The equipment used in iRacing, a virtual racing simulation that NASCAR partnered with for the series, varies in complexity but generally includes a computer equipped with a steering wheel, pedals, and high-speed internet connection. More complicated setups include a motion simulator, which can cost tens of thousands of dollars. Such simulators feature a cockpit with a seat that moves in coordination with the graphical output on the screen and integrates the steering wheel, pedals, and shifter. Some integrate the use of a VR headset for a fully immersive experience (NASCAR 2020).

VR headsets are the current evolution of Wheatstone's stereoscope. The stereoscopic images delivered are no longer fixed. Sensors keep track of what direction the head is facing, and the view inside the headset reflects what one would see in the real environment. Headphones are incorporated to provide convincing sound. VR goggles and headsets are becoming more and more accessible, with consumer-grade products at every price point. However, one area of VR is still maturing: haptics (Kuchera 2016). *Haptics* refers to technology that imparts the sense of touch. Although not new, haptic technology is set to become more sophisticated in coming years, with many current and future applications. For example, a smartphone vibrates to let you know that someone is calling or to give you real feedback when you push an imaginary button. In a video gaming system, the controller rumbles on impact when a football player makes a tackle or a car runs off the road. In the case of teledildonics, sexual partners can engage with each other from a distance by applying a remotely controlled pleasurable device to one or more partners. Other, cutting-edge applications of haptics include precision control of remote robots, such as in remote, robotic surgery (Hutson 2018). Engineers are working to take haptics to the next level; rather than simple vibrations, haptics of the future will be as real and varied as the surfaces and objects around us.

By integrating various senses, VR devices such as headsets and motion simulators re-create reality, but with one important difference: the reality being re-created is usually substantially different from the reality of the person experiencing it. What does VR provide that base reality cannot? In some cases, it is a matter of safety; for example, a pilot practicing in a flight simulator before an upcoming flight to an unfamiliar airport or a gamer wanting to experience war without the pain or discomfort of the real thing. Other times, it is a matter of practicality, such as an astronaut training for a mission or NASCAR going virtual during a pandemic. It can also be a matter of access, such as someone engaging with their favorite adult film star. The promise of VR is usually a combination of these and other driving factors, but regardless of the motivation for use, can the possibilities that VR offers be too much to resist?

Addiction vs. Nonpathological Use

Transhumanism

Transhumanism can be boiled down to the drive to become superhuman via means of augmentation. From that frame of view, we can draw at least two parallels to understand what an addiction to transhumanism may look like: performance-enhancing drugs and cosmetic surgery. Perhaps the most notorious performance-enhancing drugs are the anabolic androgenic steroids (AAS). AAS are derivatives of testosterone that promote protein synthesis and growth of muscle cells. They are used therapeutically in cases of testosterone deficiency or wasting due to chronic illness. In those instances, they are administered at physiological doses. In the case of recreational use, however, they are administered in supraphysiological doses, and the effects are often superhuman. AAS are widely used in bodybuilding to create comic book–like musculature. On playing fields and in gyms, they allow athletes to hit more home runs, run faster, hit harder, and lift more weight. At the beach, they help men and women attract mates with apparent virility. But are AAS addictive?

One of the earliest medicinal uses of exogenous testosterone was for the treatment of depression (Altschule and Tillotson 1948). This therapeutic indication has since fallen out of favor, but the use of testosterone for depression is still debated today (Walther et al. 2019). Although not intoxicating or euphoria-inducing, testosterone administration is known to cause the release of serotonin and promote neuroplasticity, and AAS are believed to cause dependence in a minority of users (Kanayama et al. 2010). They can also cause a withdrawal syndrome, and rats have been shown to self-administer AAS to the point of death (Kanayama et al. 2009). AAS dependence is associated with conduct disorder, antisocial personality disorder, and likely deficits in impulse control, as well as body dysmorphic disorder with muscle dysmorphia (Kanayama et al. 2009). Combining these elements and presupposing their application to transhumanism, we can begin to paint a picture of who might be susceptible to an unhealthy fixation with transhuman modifications: someone who perceives a deficit in themselves as compared with others, someone with poor impulse control, and perhaps someone who seeks an advantage in some form of competitive arena.

Whereas AAS involves the ingestion or administration of hormones, cosmetic surgery can show us the factors associated with unhealthy attempts at self-enhancement through a more complex form of modification as is seen in transhuman body modifications. The desire for cosmetic procedures is frequently motivated by either unhappiness with one's perception of some aspect of appearance or a belief that one's happiness will improve with some enhancement or modification. Certainly, some people experience improved subjective well-being after a cosmetic procedure. However, for others, cosmetic procedures can be troublesome. Such individuals have such a severe distortion in perception that they may never be happy, even after multiple revisions of the same procedure, exposing them to potentially increased risk of surgical complications (Ericksen and Billick 2012). Again, this suggests that transhuman enhancements may pose a risk for individuals with body dysmorphia or similar perceived deficiencies. Some research has shown an association between breast augmentation and suicide. The causes of this association remain unclear but are theorized to include mood disorders and personality disorders (Sansone and Sansone 2007). It will be curious to see which forms of transhuman augmentation are associated with poorer health outcomes such as suicide.

Positive Aspects of Transhumanism

The benefit to society of transhumanism cannot be overstated. In the case of Neil Harbisson, his transhuman modification relieved him of color blindness. A child with a smartphone has the world's knowledge at her fingertips regardless of whether that information is in a library or the wilderness. However, that fountain of knowledge is throttled by the speed of her thumbs; imagine interfacing internet access and a search engine directly with the brain, no button to click, no haptic input required. Such an advancement, which may be inevitable, could lead to untold acceleration of human progress.

Consider the potential health benefits of transhuman technology: a heart that does not fail, a constantly running internal dialysis machine or an artificial kidney, or direct input into neurological organization, brainwave patterns, and neurotransmitter balance. Elon Musk's Neuralink aims to create a brain/machine interface that could potentially mend any neurological deficit, such as restoring eyesight, curing paraplegia, and even making individuals more capable than they were before their injury. Pushed to the extreme, transhuman endeavors may lead to a truly posthuman existence: a consciousness that does not rely on a biological host at all. The tricky thing about the positive aspects of transhumanism is the subjective nature of positivity. Barring a mass extinction, the moral debates of science fiction will play out in fact.

Artificial Intelligence Addiction

It is difficult to imagine what addiction in the context of AI would look like. Several of the criteria for addiction presuppose a certain standard of functioning in our world, whereas a world with mature AI is likely to look much different than that of today. How can one have impairment in occupational functioning in a future in which human employment may not exist? Can you be addicted to an AI-powered sex robot in a future in which you have the legal authority to marry that artificial person? The criteria for addiction will likely change as emerging technology disrupts current social norms in unforeseen ways.

With this in mind, we can still speculate on technology and addiction in the immediate future. One trend in AI today is personalization. Let us consider the effect of AI algorithms when applied to advertising. If you spend any appreciable amount of time looking at a product online, there is a good chance that the next time you scroll through your social media feed you will see an advertisement for that product or its competitors. You might not realize that you are also seeing advertisements for products that the algorithm predicts you might be interested in. This is the effect of AI. Without immediate human input, the algorithm predicts which items you are more likely to purchase and presents them in a way that makes you more likely to make the purchase. Perhaps you were not ready to make the purchase that night, but the next day, after your morning cup of coffee, when you are feeling motivated and hopeful about your future, you might be more likely to hand over the virtual cash.

Another way AI steers human behavior is in the entertainment arena. Media streaming services use algorithms that attempt to learn your preferences and suggest what to watch next. In some cases, the videos play automatically, leading to hours of screen time. By learning your preferences, these AI algorithms seek to increase your consumptive behavior. The sophistication and effectiveness of these algorithms are likely to advance in the coming years.

Positive Aspects of Artificial Intelligence

AI is here to stay. There is some debate among experts on whether general AI will ever be achieved, but it is hard to count against human ingenuity if it is given enough time and motivation. It is also hard to think of a technology to which AI would not be applied. The limits of AI are unknown. A machine with true intelligence could potentially be much smarter than we are and, if so, could think of technologies, solutions, cures, and all sorts of potentially beneficial ideas that we have not even fathomed.

A common fear of AI-powered machines is that they will take our jobs, but this fear may precisely hold the key to improving our lives. With machines powering the work force and producing more wealth than we have imagined, humans could be free to spend their time however they wish. The standard of living could be raised for everyone. This would, of course, upset the current socioeconomic system. Our society identifies people by their job; what will determine our status when no jobs are being done by humans? How will we distribute wealth? Will we continue to financially oppress people based on their skin color, race, and sex? How would it be justified? Would we move to a universal basic income? Would the machines be capable of emotion, and would their forced labor amount to slavery?

Virtual Reality Addiction

The concept of being addicted to VR is not new; it has been a science fiction trope for decades. Some of the other chapters in this book demonstrate what addiction to VR looks like. Much of our technology pulls us into worlds that are virtual to us. Our social media feeds transport us to exotic locations. We spend time with friends who do not know that we exist or with lovers who never see our faces. VR technology will push these experiences to the extreme. We will not just see pictures or videos of our favorite travel vlogger; we will be there with them. We will have 360° views on all axes. We will hear every sound, feel the breeze and the raindrops on our skin, and smell the flowers or the salt of the sea. We will taste the finest dish from our favorite chef. It will be possible to achieve a level of immersion so intense that we may never want to come back.

For the more immediate future, it is still possible to picture VR addiction. Afflicted individuals may spend all waking hours of the day in VR. They may be unable to stay in the "real" world for long even if they want to. The craving to escape from a boring life into exotic fantasies may be intense. They may fail out of school or miss deadlines at work. They may tune in to VR while driving or walking on the street. They may get so used to VR that they crave ever more stimulating experiences and chase after such experiences with all of their time, energy, and money. Life in the "real" world may never be the same. It may thus be easy to become addicted to VR, and VR addiction may become an epidemic, or it may become so widespread that it becomes endemic and no longer viewed as an addiction. Even more confusing, the line between the "real" and the virtual world will likely become blurred, perhaps until that line no longer exists.

Positive Aspects of Virtual Reality

VR allows us to experience things that are impossible and to experience the extreme without the threat of mortal danger. VR has already revolutionized learning and will likely continue to do so. Pilots use VR to learn new routes and approaches to foreign ports. Astronauts use it to perfect the steps of their mission or practice corrective actions. Physicians will use VR to practice procedures many times before operating on a real patient. Testing for certification will become closer to real-life scenarios. Police and military will use VR to practice navigating difficult situations. Psychiatrists will use VR for exposure therapy in PTSD, phobias, and other anxiety disorders.

VR may benefit the environment as well. It has the potential to reduce the use of disposable materials. Advertising on paper or plastic products will seem silly in comparison to the powerful experience mature VR will deliver. Someone who is learning to fly or to drive can get hours of experience without burning any fuel. VR will help push environmental causes; we will be more motivated to act when we can see, hear, smell, taste, and feel the Amazon rainforest or be among the black rhinos or the vaquitas in real time.

Treatment

Treatments for emerging technological addictions will be as diverse and patient centered as the field of addiction psychiatry is today. A biopsychosocial assessment and formulation may provide insight into the driving forces behind a person's use of a particular technology and may reveal an underlying diagnosis or comorbidity, an added benefit of which is allowing the use of an FDA-approved medication rather than relying on off-label use. In the case of transhumanism, psychiatrists may identify the underlying motivation for pathological body modifications as they do with common addictions today. The psychodynamic drive that precipitates the pathological behavior will be explored. A cognitive-behavioral approach can help to identify underlying cognitive distortions: Is there body dysmorphia? In that case, perhaps a selective serotonin reuptake inhibitor may help. Could this person have bipolar disorder and go on sprees of consumptive activity, of which body modifications are just one part? Perhaps psychoeducation and a mood stabilizer will be the key. Does this patient experience euphoria when having procedures done? Perhaps naltrexone is indicated.

In addition to VR, what is it about the person's behavior that makes her use of VR pathological? What domain of her life is being affected? Has she lost a job or failed out of school because of spending too much time in VR landscapes? When she is away from VR, does she experience a physiological and psychological withdrawal that causes her to suffer? Is there something about her "real life" that she is trying to escape? Might she be trying to avoid an intrusive reexperiencing of a traumatic event? Are there interpersonal issues she is seeking to repress? Is there some life role she feels ill-equipped to perform and would therefore rather occupy herself elsewhere? What are these factors, and how can they be addressed practically?

In the case of unhealthy use of AI, several factors may be explored. Is this person overreliant on the use of AI because he is lonely? Could this loneliness be a smaller piece of a larger mood disorder? Could he have social anxiety disorder and be seeking an outlet that he is unable to achieve in other situations? Perhaps the opportunistic algorithms used by AI developers are causing neurotransmitter surges in individuals with an addictive propensity. Could this patient have ADHD and be susceptible to the constant source of stimulation AI can deliver? Again, the specific type of psychotherapy, medication management, and other therapeutic interventions are tailored to the patient and the circumstances.

Special Considerations

The technologies covered in this chapter are just a tiny sliver of what lies ahead. Transhumanism, AI, and VR were selected because they are established fields that are set to accelerate because the science fueling them is now maturing. Given the evolving role that these technologies play in society, it would be useful for the treating psychiatrist to be flexible and open-minded when assessing whether a patient's behavior is pathological. The hallmark of psychiatric illness is distress and impairment of functioning. Frequency of use and negative popular opinion do not in themselves define an addiction. Attitudes toward emerging technologies change, and what may seem detrimental now may prove to be crucial to the next generation.

KEY POINTS

- Transhumanism is a movement dedicated to enhancing human abilities through technology, sometimes with the goal of reaching a superhuman or posthuman state. Given the addictive potential of anabolic androgenic steroids and cosmetic surgery, transhumanism may become a new frontier of the technological addictions.

- Emerging subfields of artificial intelligence (AI) include natural language processing, such as that employed by virtual assistants that communicate with humans in their own tongues, and machine learning algorithms, which aim to equip computers with the ability to adapt and learn from their own experiences with programmer intervention.

- AI algorithms learn individuals' preferences and behavior, sway those individuals' behavior, and inherently put people at risk of having their addictive propensities exploited.

- Virtual reality (VR) technology often integrates multiple sensory inputs to create either simulated or enhanced environments for people to experience.

- Treatment of addiction to transhuman technology, AI, VR, and other emerging technologies will likely require individualized psychotherapy and medication management informed by underlying contributing factors when applicable.

Practice Questions

1. Which of the following types of technologies is most closely associated with the use of artificial neural networks and computer generalization of data?

    A. Remote surgery
    B. Augmented reality
    C. Transhumanism

D. Machine learning

E. Haptics

Answer: D.

Machine learning is a subfield of artificial intelligence (AI) that aims to enable computers to learn without human intervention, often with the use of systems known as *neural networks*. Remote surgery (A) does not require machine learning. Augmented reality (B) is a subfield of virtual reality that usually involves placing computer-generated objects in the real world. Transhumanism (C) is the use of technology to enhance human physiology. Haptics (E) focus on touch in technological interactions.

2. A 16-year-old girl is brought to your office in late July by her mother, who is concerned that her daughter is spending too much time in her room and worried that she might be depressed. The patient reports that she spends up to 10 hours per day logged into a new online virtual experience, which involves a headset with three-dimensional video and high-fidelity audio and allows users to create characters and interact with other players from around the world. She sleeps in late and stays up until dawn so that she can play along with her friends from Europe. She says that she enjoys the experience because she feels that she can be herself. In school, she gets As on her examinations but often gets marked down for not participating in class. She does not go to parties, even though she is often invited, and does not get along with girls her age because they are so judgmental. She wishes she had more friends, which makes her feel depressed.

    What is the most likely diagnosis?

    A. Virtual reality addiction

    B. Internet gaming disorder

    C. Major depressive disorder

    D. Bipolar disorder

    E. Social anxiety disorder

Answer: E.

This patient is unable to speak in school despite often knowing the answers. She dreads going to parties or other social outings and views her peers as being judgmental. Through the relative anonymity of this new virtual reality (VR) experience, she is able to overcome her cognitive distortions of constantly being judged and can socialize with other people, which she desperately craves. Social anxiety disorder can be a crippling illness that can easily lead to depression (C) or substance use. Although the patient identifies as feeling depressed, has disrupted sleep, does not leave home or socialize, and to her mom appears as though she has lost interest in life, the more prominent issue hinted at by the patient is social anxiety. It is quite likely that if her anxiety were better managed, her mood would improve.

VR addiction (A) is not a DSM diagnosis. This patient spends all day engaged in her VR experience; however, she presents during the summer when there is no school. There is no mention of her not meeting other obligations, and she does not appear to suffer from her VR use. She is an A student, and to the extent that her presentation overlaps with an addiction, it is likely better explained by her social anxiety. The same logic applies to internet gaming disorder (B). People with social anxiety disorder may spend many hours playing massively multiplayer online roleplaying games or other internet-based games. This patient reports staying up late at night, and individuals with anxiety disorders may answer affirmatively to inquiries of racing thoughts and irritability. They can also appear distracted to others. However, bipolar disorder (D) can be ruled out by the absence of discrete hypomanic or manic episodes. This patient would likely report that these symptoms represent her baseline mood and behavior.

3. Melissa is reluctantly brought to the clinic by her husband, who is concerned about her behavior. Every evening, she spends several hours in the bathroom looking in the mirror. During this time, she is often picking at her skin, posing in the mirror, and scrolling through social media. She often makes self-deprecating remarks about her appearance and seeks reassurance from her husband. She has accumulated more than $20,000 in credit card debt over the past 2 years. Most of the money has been spent on skin creams, beauty products, and supplements, as well as payment plans for several surgical procedures, including breast augmentation, gluteal augmentation, rhytidectomy, botulinum toxin injections, and lip fillers. She also had a near field communication chip implanted on the dorsum of her hand, with subdermal light-emitting diodes and several microsensors that measure electrolytes, volatile compounds, and the hydration status of her skin. The chip connects with a subscription-based service that recommends individualized skin-care products on a weekly basis.

   Which of these medications would be most indicated for Melissa?

A. Valproic acid
B. Gabapentin
C. Methylphenidate
D. Fluoxetine
E. Olanzapine

Answer: D.

Melissa's clinical presentation is a classic case of body dysmorphic disorder with the integration of new and emerging technologies that will factor in our lives. The technological applications discussed in the question are based on ones available on the market today. The other medications on the list (A, B, C, and E) could potentially be useful for individuals with an unhealthy use of technology, based on their circumstances and physiology. In this case, with a diagnosis of body dysmorphic disorder, a selective serotonin reuptake inhibitor is an excellent first-line treatment because her potentially unhealthy use of technology is at least partially secondary to a condition that responds well to that class of medication.

Resources for Clinicians, Patients, and Families

Common Sense (commonsensemedia.org): Nonprofit organization that provides research-backed information, education, and advocacy for parents and educators, aimed ensuring digital well-being for children.

The Psychiatrists Guide Podcast (https://www.thepsychiatristsguide.com): Podcast that covers a wide range of topics, including emerging technologies in psychiatry, cohosted by Rafael Coira, M.D., J.D., and James Sherer, M.D., two of this book's authors.

References

Altschule MD, Tillotson KJ: The use of testosterone in the treatment of depressions. N Engl J Med 239(27):1036–1038, 1948 18103557

Aschburner S: Coronavirus pandemic causes NBA to suspend season after player tests positive, NBA, March 12, 2020. Available at: https://www.nba.com/article/2020/03/11/coronavirus-pandemic-causes-nba-suspend-season. Accessed April 15, 2020.

BBC News: Computer AI passes Turing test in 'world first.' BBC News, June 9, 2014. Available at: https://www.bbc.com/news/technology-27762088. Accessed April 8, 2020.

Brennan C: When what you see is not in colour. The Irish Times, May 27, 2008. Available at: https://www.irishtimes.com/news/health/when-what-you-see-is-not-in-colour-1.1215430. Accessed April 8, 2020.

Cyborg Arts: Neil Harbisson. Cyborgarts.com, 2020. Available at: https://www.cyborgarts.com/neil-harbisson. Accessed July 31, 2020.

Ericksen WL, Billick SB: Psychiatric issues in cosmetic plastic surgery. Psychiatr Q 83(3):343–352, 2012 22252848

Garbade M: A simple introduction to natural language processing. Becoming Human, October 15, 2018. Available at: https://becominghuman.ai/a-simple-introduction-to-natural-language-processing-ea66a1747b32. Accessed April 22, 2020.

Harris J: What is machine learning? Brookings, October 4, 2018. Available at: https://www.brookings.edu/research/what-is-machine-learning. Accessed April 22, 2020.

Hutson M: Here's what the future of haptic technology looks (or rather, feels) like. Smithsonian Magazine, December 28, 2018

Kanayama G, Brower KJ, Wood RI, et al: Anabolic-androgenic steroid dependence: an emerging disorder. Addiction 104(12):1966–1978, 2009 19922565

Kanayama G, Hudson JI, Pope HG Jr: Illicit anabolic-androgenic steroid use. Horm Behav 58(1):111–121, 2010 19769977

Kuchera B: The complete guide to virtual reality in 2016. Polygon, January 15, 2016. Available at: https://www.polygon.com/2016/1/15/10772026/virtual-reality-guide-oculus-google-cardboard-gear-vr. Accessed May 5, 2020.

NASCAR: eNASCAR iRacing Pro Invitational Series. Enascar.com, 2020. Available at: https://www.enascar.com/iracing-pro-invitational-series. Accessed July 31, 2020.

Sansone RA, Sansone LA: Cosmetic surgery and psychological issues. Psychiatry (Edgmont) 4(12):65–68, 2007 20436768

Stix M: World's first cyborg wants to hack your body. CNN Business, January 7, 2016. Available at: https://www.cnn.com/2014/09/02/tech/innovation/cyborg-neil-harbisson-implant-antenna/index.html. Accessed April 8, 2020.

2045 Strategic Social Initiative: About us. 2045.com, 2020. Available at: http://2045.com/about. Accessed July 31, 2020.

Virtual Reality Society: History of Virtual Reality. VRS.org.uk, 2020. Available at: https://www.vrs.org.uk/virtual-reality/history.html. Accessed July 31, 2020.

Walther A, Breidenstein J, Miller R: Association of testosterone treatment with alleviation of depressive symptoms in men: a systematic review and meta-analysis. JAMA Psychiatry 76(1):31–40, 2019 30427999

Warwick K, Gasson M, Hutt B, et al: The application of implant technology for cybernetic systems. Arch Neurol 60(10):1369–1373, 2003 14568806

Index

Page numbers printed in **boldface** type refer to tables and figures.